PRAIS
By I

MW00596850

Dr. Scherger brings the wisdom and experience gained over 30 years of conventional medical practice and physician education into the newly enlightened realm of functional medicine. His work is all the more important, as he has lived and breathed both sides of the healthcare world, now bringing his unique perspectives into reviewing some of the more important books and ideas he has surveyed since beginning his new functional medicine journey.

-- William Davis, MD
Author of the *Wheat Belly* books

I read your book with great interest. Very nice, easy to read piece with personal learnings and commentary. The information describing the impact of a diet (healthy and unhealthy) on the gut microbiome, the hippocampus and select chronic conditions is most interesting and fascinating.

-- Mary Madison
MM Consulting

JOSEPH E. SCHERGER, MD, MPH

Lean and Fit
A Doctor's Journey to Healthy Nutrition and Greater Wellness

Revised and Expanded

JOSEPH E. SCHERGER, MD, MPH

MEDICAL DISCLAIMER
The information presented in this book is the result of many years of practice experience and clinical research by the author. The information in this book, by necessity, is of a general nature and not a substitute for an evaluation or treatment by a competent medical specialist. If you believe you are in need of medical intervention, please see a medical practitioner as soon as possible.

DEDICATIONS

To my mentor physicians, William Davis,
David Perlmutter, Mark Hyman, Terry Wahls,
Gerard Mullin, Robynne Chutkin, David Ludwig,
Robert Lustig and my partner in practice
(and personal physician) Hessam Mahdavi,
all champions of nutrition for better health.

To Robert Atkins, Jeff Volek and Stephen Phinney for
advancing the science of low carbohydrate nutrition.

To Daniel Lieberman at Harvard and
Justin and Erica Sonnenburg at Stanford
for teaching us about the human body.

ACKNOWLEDGMENTS

To my team of Helen Searing and my son Adrian Scherger
for making this book special and getting the message of
Lean and Fit to a wide audience through
www.leanandfitlife.com

To my friend and patient Barbara Rogers for her great
recipes, found in the Appendix and on our website
www.leanandfitlife.com and on her website,
www.itsanograinerlife.com.

LEAN AND FIT

CONTENTS

Conclusions   77

Appendices   81-102

References   103

About the Author   114

PREFACE

Why do we keep poisoning ourselves? We do not know any better. Sure we think we do. It must be the sugary beverages, or the supersizing of french fries at fast food restaurants. Those are problems but they are not the big picture. The real cause of the poisoning that has made most of us overweight or obese, with a staggering burden of diseases, is a toxic food environment of high glycemic carbohydrates and inflammatory proteins. As the famed evolutionary biologist from Harvard, Daniel Lieberman, has written, cultural evolution has given us a diet and lifestyle that do not match our evolutionary bodies, and these result in a large burden of chronic disease.

I know this sounds extreme. Aren't bread and cookies and cupcakes and brownies and bagels and ice cream normal foods? No they are not. Look around. The majority of people are seriously overweight and more than 1 in 3 are obese. Diabetes, type 1 and 2, do not need to happen. The auto-immune diseases, from lupus to rheumatoid arthritis to hypothyroidism do not need to happen. Autism and multiple sclerosis and Parkinson's disease and Alzheimer's disease do not need to happen. Acne and rosacea do not need to happen. High blood pressure and high cholesterol do not need to happen. Acid reflux and irritable bowel syndrome do not need to happen. All are diseases of malnutrition.

We evolved to eat the foods nature gives us – vegetables, fruits, nuts, seeds, fish and meat from animals fed on the land. We have never had such a variety and abundance of these foods available. Yet we have created foods that harm us such as breads and other flour based foods and sweets. Hospitals continue to serve unhealthy food. We entice doctors and medical students to come to meetings by serving pizza or bagels. We reward our police and ambulance drivers by giving them doughnuts. We celebrate by having parties that serve cake. The inconvenient truth, as this book will describe, is that these pleasurable foods are hurting us in very serious ways.

So much has been written in the last year that I am compelled to publish a second edition of this book. Also, based on your feedback I have added material that makes this book more complete, such as a listing of "Superfoods" and some discussion of supplements. I have continued to write articles on healthy nutrition and lifestyle and those are included here.

In the Preface to the first edition I stated that "The biology of human health is poorly understood." After receiving training in the emerging field of Functional Medicine in July 2016, I realize we know much more about our biology. We have deep knowledge in what makes us healthy and sick. The new material in this book reflects much of that information. We still have much to learn.

We are sustained by what we eat yet what constitutes the right healthy diet is highly controversial and keeps changing. We recently discovered a new "organ system", the human microbiome, and that may turn out to be the most important of all.

This book is about my health, a family doctor with a career long interest in preventive medicine as much as my interest in disease. As someone who has always strived to be healthy, at age 63, much of what I thought was healthy nutrition has changed. As I used new knowledge to change my nutrition, my health went from good to great. My journey to healthy nutrition and greater wellness continues and I plan to stay on that path for as long as I live. That may be longer then the lifespan we are accustomed to!

I share this journey, and some of the articles I have written, in hopes that it will help you become healthier. Everyone's life is a journey and we make many choices along the way. Far better health and longevity with a greater healthspan are within our reach. We are designed to be lean and fit, yet there are powerful forces working against us, especially in the United States. But knowledge is power and hopefully you will find some of my journey useful as you navigate your way to better health.

Like the first edition, this second edition is short and to the point. Readers have told me the two best things about my book are that it tells a personal story and is not too long. This book can be read in one sitting. I include new articles for you to digest or skip over. Be sure to study the Appendices, since some of the most important information is there. My thanks to friend and patient Barbara Rogers for her recipes!

My efforts with *Lean and Fit* will move to a new website, www.leanandfitlife.com. There I will provide updated information, welcome reader input and suggestions, and will make available personalized professional advice and coaching for you to thrive on your own journey to healthy nutrition and greater wellness.

You only get one body, take care of it!

Joseph E. Scherger, MD, MPH
October 2016

PART 1: 63 YEARS OF MOSTLY GOOD HEALTH

I came from a family with a strong health orientation in the small town of Delphos, Ohio in the Northwestern part of the state that resembles the flat farmlands of the Midwest. My home town of 7000 people was surrounded by corn fields and wheat fields. My father was president of the local bank and spent much of his time lending money to farmers. Our family kept an eye out for health news and I was raised on a lot of whole wheat bread and cow's milk. My parents reverted to skim milk when the low fat products were promoted.

Both my parents lived into their early 90s, so I have good genes. My father suffered near the end of his life with Parkinson's disease and eventually the dementia that accompanies that dreadful neurodegenerative illness. He died a shadow of his former self. My mother suffered from gallbladder disease and died two years after my father mainly to join him in heaven.

Growing up my favorite food was bacon and I would always order 10 strips from an obliging mother who lived by the philosophy "feed them what they will eat". In high school I had two hot dogs almost every night before bed with a glass of milk. I was not a good athlete in the three team sports, football, basketball and baseball, but I stayed lean and fit riding a bicycle most everywhere and playing golf and tennis.

My big nuisance health problem was acne. It started like most teenagers at puberty but it did not want to go away as I became an adult. I was embarrassed often in medical school with big zits in my 20s. Finally in my 50s the pimples receded but I developed an adult form of acne, rosacea on and around my nose. In my early 60s I was applying an antibiotic gel on and around my nose twice a day until I discovered what was causing the problem, but that story is in the next part of this book.

I was healthier at 30 than I was at 20. At age 20 I was studying hard in college in order to get to medical school and I got very little exercise. I never become overweight in my 20s but I had limited muscle strength and by today's standards would be called a nerd. In my late 20s finishing my medical training in family medicine and public health, I joined the running craze that developed in the 1970s. I started my medical practice in the college town of Davis, California and my neighbor was a runner. He invited me to join him in the Runner's World 12 week training schedule to run a marathon. I was already running about 30 minutes on most days so I was ripe for this effort.

Our first race was the Bay to Breakers 8 mile run in San Francisco that was so much fun I was hooked. Our first marathon in 1979, me at age 29, was the President's Cup in San Francisco that was held only once because the police said no way they would block that much traffic again. We started on Treasure Island in San Francisco Bay and ran over the Bay Bridge to the Embarcadero. We ran by all the piers and through the Presidio and went back and forth over the Golden Gate Bridge. The 26.2 miles ended in Golden Gate Park. My neighbor was quite fast and made his goal of less than 3 hours to qualify for Boston. We ran three marathons together over three years and with his fast pace inspiration I finished them between 3:15 and 3:30, despite getting only water along the way and hitting the "wall" around 20 miles as my muscles ran out of energy. At age 30 I was lean and fit weighing 155 pounds at 5 feet 11 inches. I had a 32-inch waist. I felt like the statue of David.

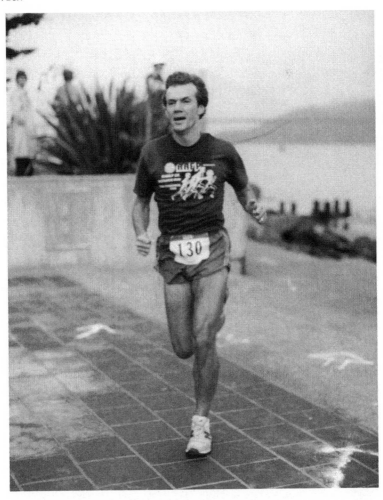

In 1982 my neighbor moved away and I became very busy with my medical practice. My running tapered off to the occasional 5k. By age 46 my weight was 192 pounds, my peak, and not good. My total cholesterol was 211 and my HDL (good cholesterol) was only 37.

Despite my parents' longevity, heart disease runs in our family and I was at risk. I faced the decision to go on a statin or lose the weight. One of my two sons inspired me to become a runner again and do marathons. That seemed the healthy choice. I also cut out some of the fat in my diet such as salad dressings and butter on bread, decisions I would not make today.

By age 63 I had run 30 marathons and had even started running ultramarathons at age 61 after reading the life altering book, *Born to Run* by Christopher McDougall. My weight came down to 180 on this plan and my cholesterol dropped to 175 with HDL cholesterol of 52. No statin for me and it shows how exercise and weight loss can lower total cholesterol and raise the HDL. Oddly my waistline was still 36 inches. At 180 pounds I was a heavy runner.

At age 57 I developed another health problem. I became mildly hypothyroid, a common autoimmune problem. I knew something was not quite right. I felt a little sluggish, my running became slower and it was hard to lose weight. Sure enough my TSH was above the normal range. That corrected with a modest dose of levothyroxine. Why had I developed this problem with no family history of hypothyroidism? I would find out why later.

I am also a medical writer and my first book, *Forty Years in Family Medicine,* is a collection of articles I have written over my career. What follows is an article summarizing a healthy lifestyle first published in 2000 and updated for today. A healthy lifestyle can be summarized in eight simple phrases: Eat Right, Be Active, Manage Stress, Be Happy, Have Purpose, Don't Smoke, Be Safe and Sleep Well. Each two word combination is a pillar of good health.

Living a Healthy Lifestyle

The rules are simple. They have been known for a long time. They are more important than ever.

A century ago, living a healthy lifestyle might not have given much assurance for a long and healthy life. If you acquired a serious skin infection or appendicitis, chances were you would die. We have conquered many of the causes of premature death that plagued mankind prior to the twentieth century. Now in the twenty-first century, good health and a long life are more than ever a choice.

Genetics, infections, accidents, or cancers may end life early for some, but lifestyle factors loom as the leading cause of premature death. Promoting a healthy lifestyle must now become a principal focus for anyone wanting to live a long, happy and healthy life.

Despite the extravagant claims of supplement manufacturers, good health does not come in a bottle. A "fountain of youth" craze seems to come over the population periodically, a hope for simple external solutions to what is an internal issue. The 1890s were the decade of patent medicines, with a proliferation of nostrums promising good health. Curiously, we see a similar public fascination with unproved medications today as pharmacies all over the country devote expanding amounts of square footage to nutritional supplements that promise various health benefits. Truth and common sense usually prevail, and I suspect this current preoccupation will pass. Perhaps then we will have a more receptive audience for the timeless rules of healthful living. These rules are straightforward – we heard most of them first from our parents. These eight rules are stated simply, but are hard for some people to follow. If following any of these is hard for you, get help. Your life depends on it.

Eat Right

A healthy lifestyle begins with nutrition. You are what you eat is an age old expression that is just as true today. We are a living organism completely dependent on what we eat. What happens to our body is more dependent on our nutrition than any other factor.

Eating right seems more confusing than ever. Back in 2000 I was promoting a low fat, high fiber diet as recommended by the American Heart Association. I love starting off the day with a healthy breakfast and back then it was a high fiber cereal. No more. As you will read in more detail in this book, the science of nutrition has progressed and processed carbohydrates, including whole grains, are the cause of many health problems.

After years of thinking modern society could improve health by processing foods, we realize that eating the foods of nature is the healthiest choice. Our evolutionary body is incredibly complex and evolved over millions of years to thrive on the foods of nature – vegetables, nuts, seeds, fruit, wild meat and fish. Most of this book will explore healthy eating in more detail, and the suggested reading is a treasure trove of vital information.

Be Active

The evidence supporting the health benefits of physical activity and the consequences of inactivity are so compelling that this rule rises to number two. Many adults have become more physically active in the last two decades, contributing to a decline in heart disease. However, a growing number of young people are not physically active, and obesity among children is on the rise. Work at home and on the job is less physically demanding today, and conscious choices must be made to walk and get other forms of exercise. Recent research shows that all physical activity counts and its benefits are cumulative. As we make time for exercise in our own busy lives, we should regularly inquire about our family and friends activity levels and encourage them to become physically active. Families and social groups that exercise together thrive together!

Part 2 of this book covers physical fitness in greater detail.

Manage Stress

Stress is a major cause of disease, even life threatening problems such as heart disease and cancer. Modern life is complicated and many people find themselves in highly stressful work or home situations. Making adjustments to reduce stress is important but may not always be an option.

Managing stress is a skill that everyone should learn. There are many options such as meditation, relaxation exercises, and having a "spa day". Taking charge of your life and making adjustments are very important to your survival. One patient taught me AMTD (Attitude Makes the Difference). Some people have the hardiness to turn distress in to eustress that is stress that you actually enjoy. You can enjoy stress more if you have control over the situation and living a life of your choice.

Be Happy

I am not suggesting a false sense of bliss, but having a positive outlook has many health benefits. My first "patient" in this regard was my freshman college roommate. To him, life was a joyless, uphill struggle. He grew up on Long Island, the son of an industrial assembly line worker. I am proud to say that now with persistent encouragement from me and others he became a remarkably healthy and optimistic school superintendent.

Depression is a leading cause of disease and disability worldwide. Mental health is critically important to overall health. In any way we can, we should model and promote positivity.

Have Purpose

George Engel suggested a biopsychosocial model for medicine in the 1970s. The body, mind and social connections should all be healthy. The growing evidence regarding spirituality and health suggests a connection. Purpose or having a higher meaning to your life than mere existence is important for overall health. Explore this dimension with family and friends. Become part of social groups that provide real meaning to your life and enjoy the health benefits.

Don't Smoke

Smoking tobacco continues to be the leading cause of premature disease and death in the U.S. and most of the world. Being healthy means not consuming things that harm the body. Tobacco, like other substances, is addicting and if you smoke, get the help you need to stop. Your brain will crave what you are addicted to, even sugar, and overcoming such addictions is a crucial step to a healthy lifestyle.

Be Safe

Accidents loom large as a preventable cause of death, especially among the young. Wear seat belts and bicycle helmets, use infant car seats, and drive safely. Components of home safety such as smoke detectors, safe appliances and electrical wiring, gun locks, and fences around pools may be lifesaving. Accidents are the fifth leading cause of death in the U.S. Any effort you can make to prevent accidents is time well spent.

Sleep Well

We should be spending between one third and one quarter of our lives in sound sleep. Poor sleep habits are common and the health consequences are becoming better known. Most fibromyalgia patients improve with better sleep. Drowsiness kills on highways. We train our children to sleep, sometimes a challenging task, but as adults we often fall into poor sleep habits and lack a "parent" to set us straight again. Without restful sleep, about 7 hours a night for most, health suffers and we become dangerous. Do everything you can to get restful sleep without medications, except for the natural sleep hormone Melatonin needed by many seniors.

For updates on living a healthy lifestyle visit www.leanandfitlife.com and be part of the discussion and coaching.

PART 2: DO YOU LIVE IN THE KINGDOM OF THE FIT?

Being fit is not difficult. I often tell patients there are two kingdoms in the world: the kingdom of the fit and the kingdom of the out of shape. In which kingdom do you live? The admission ticket to the kingdom of the fit is just 5 hours a week of focused physical activity. There are 168 hours in a week. That leaves 163 hours a week to do everything else. If you do not live in the kingdom of the fit, why not? Your health and your life depend on it.

Exercise can take many forms. They are usually divided into aerobic or movement exercise that makes your heart rate and breathing increase, and anaerobic exercise that builds muscle strength. Every week a fit person engages in both.

There are many options for aerobic exercise. Walking may be the most common type and is the preferred exercise in middle age and for seniors. Walking should be as brisk as your health and fitness allows.

If you are young or if your hips and knees are healthy, you may safely engage in jogging or running. Contrary to popular belief, jogging and running do not wear out your knees and hips. The contrary is true. At Stanford a longitudinal study was done of people in their 50s followed for 20 years. The regular runners actually developed less knee arthritis (20%) compared with the non-runners (36%). Running on healthy knees actually allows the cartilage in the knees, the cushions that go between the large bones, to grow rather than shrink. This cartilage growth may be helped by taking a combination of glucosamine, chondroitin and MSM, one of the few supplements I take.

There are many other forms of aerobic exercise such as cycling, swimming, rowing, and activities in a fitness center such as the treadmill, elliptical machines and stair masters. Choose what you enjoy and you are more likely to stay with it. Do aerobic exercise for at least thirty minutes 3-5 days a week.

Cross train your aerobic activity with strength training appropriate to your age, gender and overall health. Have a routine to strengthen your upper body, core (abdomen and back) and lower body. I recommend at least one appointment with a personal trainer to get your routine. Do strength training for at least 20 minutes a minimum of three days a week.

A combination of weekly aerobic and anaerobic exercise for 5 hours a week or more should be as important to your schedule as eating and sleeping. Dynamic or movement stretching accomplishes some of both types of exercise. Tai chi, yoga, Pilates and other stretching routines are good and preferred by many. I especially recommend the routines of former ballerina and fitness instructor Miranda Esmonde-White in her book, *Aging Backwards* (2014).

In addition to focused exercise, look for opportunities to be physically active in your daily routine. Walk more by parking farther away from your destination, or walk or bicycle to work or other activities. Take the stairs whenever possible rather than the elevator. I get an average of 8 flights of stairs every work day doing this. This helps me with hill climbing in my trail runs.

I have been a long distance runner since my 20s and am fortunate to have very healthy legs at age 66. I published the following article in 2000 and is updated here.

Why Do I Run?

	1997	2000	2016
Weight:	190 lb	178 lb	162 lb
Total Cholesterol:	211	160	152
HDL Cholesterol:	37	51	69

Those were my numbers at different times in my life. What made the difference was 10-20 miles a week of running and a healthy diet. Between 1997 and 2000 I returned to running after a 15 year hiatus and made modest dietary changes, what I thought was healthy at the time. In 2013, after reading *Wheat Belly* and the other books cited here, I cut out grains, excess sugars and moderated my alcohol intake and quickly lost the extra weight and my lipid numbers became ideal and remain so in 2016.

My weight and lipid numbers in 1997, at age 47, frightened me. Too many restaurant dinners and too little time for physical activity were taking their toll. One of my sons challenged me to get back in shape and run a marathon with him. He reminded me that I'd run three marathons when he was a young child. That was just the push I needed.

I learned from *Galloway's Book on Running* to train for a marathon by running just 20 to 25 miles a week. Such a regimen accommodated my busy life as a doctor. After just four months of training, my weight was down and my lipids much better. Since the first marathon I ran with my son, on Father's Day in 1998, I have run thirty-three more by age 66, and fifteen ultramarathon trail runs (ten 50k and five 50 miles). Today I feel younger and better than I did when I turned 40.

The benefits of regular physical activity are well documented. Going from unfit to fit reduces all-cause mortality by as much as 44%. Besides reducing the risk of cardiovascular disease, regular physical activity reduces colon cancer risk, improves glucose control, increases insulin sensitivity, and lowers blood pressure. Recent studies suggest it may stimulate the growth of brain cells, thus reducing the risk of memory loss.

Research has shown that even moderate physical activity helps. We should promote to our inactive family and friends to include more physical activity in their daily routines – walking more, taking the stairs, doing things by hand. Structured exercise is the second step, and we should make time for it may be just as vital to your health as eating and sleeping.

The mental health benefits of exercise are as important as the physical effects. The same son who encouraged me to resume running later suffered a near-fatal auto accident on January 1, 2000. Running helped me deal with the stress of his tragedy and the hard work of helping him recover. Now he runs for his own mental and physical health.

Being sedentary carries its own risks: It contributes substantially to the likelihood of coronary heart disease, Type 2 diabetes, and colon cancer – all potentially fatal. In 1992, the American Heart Association named physical inactivity as an independent risk factor for cardiovascular disease. Recent evidence shows that lack of cardiorespiratory fitness may be more of a health risk than obesity.

Promoting regular physical activity is a challenge worth taking on. We need to individualize our advice as people have their own ways of – and reasons for – being active. I do not entirely enjoy running marathons. They are painful, but the pain is quickly forgotten, replaced by a sense of accomplishment. Sharing my marathon experiences with others may help them find their own motivation for making exercise a part of their lives.

PART 3: DROP THE WHEAT AND LOSE THE WEIGHT

I am avid listener of recorded books. There has been a book in my car continuously for the last 30 years. First it was Books on Tape and I went through many boxes. Then it became CDs. Now I use *Audible.com*, a subsidiary of Amazon and the books are download into my iPad and are Bluetoothed into my car's sound system. I listen to all kinds of nonfiction where I think I can learn something. I am a history buff and learn a lot from good biographies of people I admire. I do enjoy the occasional novel. With *Audible.com* I get a "Daily Deal" in my morning email offering a book that day for less than $5. One day in September 2013, at age 63, the Daily Deal was *Wheat Belly* by Dr. William Davis.

I studied nutrition when getting my Masters in Public Health (MPH) at the University of Washington in 1978 and followed the latest nutrition recommendations carefully. I counseled and practiced a diet of low fat and high fiber from whole grains. *Wheat Belly* looked interesting.

Good books can change your life and *Wheat Belly* did just that. With great detail backed up by good scientific references, Dr. Davis described the two health problems caused by modern wheat. First is the heavy carbohydrate load and it is clear that the heavy intake of carbohydrates is the main problem behind the overweight and obesity epidemic. Carbohydrates drive hunger and when we ingest more of them we eat more. The epidemic of overweight and obesity coincided with the development of the low fat food industry. Low fat means more carbohydrates. Robert Atkins was right after all back in the 1970s and the American Heart Association and the American Diabetes Association got it wrong.

The second big health problem with wheat is the inflammatory proteins. These proteins found in all grains appear to cause a wide range of health problems. The most well-known of the inflammatory proteins is the gluten complex in wheat, barley and rye. Gluten is not a single protein but a complex of proteins mainly consisting of gliadin and gutenin. Gliadin is the most inflammatory. Celiac disease is an extreme form of gluten intolerance and those who suffer cannot ingest even trace amounts of wheat. However, it appears that we all may suffer from what is being called non-celiac gluten sensitivity.

I listened to this book not just once but twice and then ordered 15 copies. To be sure I learned everything I could from this book I read it in print form and gave the others out to friends and recommended it for patients.

I gave up all foods made with flour and changes began to happen quickly. I started losing weight without dieting almost like magic. What is amazing is that when you give up these high glycemic foods your hunger drive almost disappears. After a breakfast I will describe later, I was not hungry by lunch time and would eat less. A smaller dinner of a good entrée and vegetables was totally satisfying. No more food cravings.

In addition, by going off gluten my rosacea went away! I learned from Chapter 12 of *Wheat Belly* that my acne for so many years and later rosacea were caused by the inflammatory effects of gluten. Gluten also set me up for the autoimmune problem of hypothyroidism. I will be on thyroid medication the rest of my life thanks to wheat.

As I made this rapid health transformation I was inspired to read more books. I followed *Wheat Belly* with *Grain Brain* by neurologist and nutritionist Dr. David Perlmutter. Perlmutter describes how elevated blood sugar from grains and sweets accelerates brain atrophy and increases the progression to dementia. From him I learned the importance of getting my fasting blood sugar to less than 90 and getting my HbA1c, a test for control of diabetes, to the lowest level possible. HbA1c is a measurement of the average blood sugar over 3 months by looking at how much sugar coats our red blood cells that live in our body for about 3 months. The lower the blood sugar the sharper our mind. In addition, the inflammatory protein complex gluten has a toxic effect on the brain and most likely causes neurodegenerative disease such as multiple sclerosis and Alzheimer's disease.

Health and longevity are not just about a great lipid panel and avoiding dementia. Cancer looms as a cause of about one third of premature deaths. An academic nutritionist and cancer epidemiologist, Colin Campbell at

Cornell, was frustrated that his more than 400 scientific papers contained vital health information but were not known to the public. He went public with his 2006 book, *The China Study*. I read his 2013 book, *Whole: Rethinking the Science of Nutrition*. Campbell is a champion of a whole food plant based diet after finding the populations that lived all or mostly on vegetables lived healthier and longer lives, and had the lowest rates of cancer. Campbell is a hero of the vegan diet and even claims that following it carefully may help reverse some cancers. I wonder why all cancer centers do not promote a whole food plant based diet.

I wrote a collective book review of *Wheat Belly*, *Grain Brain* and *Whole* for the journal *Family Medicine* which is updated here:

Big Ideas in Nutrition: Three Books Worth Knowing

Wheat Belly. William Davis, M.D. Rodale. 2011.

Grain Brain. David Perlmutter, M.D. Little, Brown and Co. 2013.

Whole: Rethinking the Science of Nutrition. T. Colin Campbell, PhD, Howard Jacobson, PhD. BenBella Books. 2013.

Let food by thy medicine and medicine be thy food.
Hippocrates

Much has happened in food science since the recommended four food groups of the 1950s. With emerging evidence about heart disease caused by atherosclerosis and the role of cholesterol, low saturated fat diets were promoted. Unfortunately, many people replaced saturated fats with high glycemic carbohydrates and the overweight, obesity and type 2 diabetes epidemics took off in 1980. Robert Atkins first promoted a low carbohydrate diet in the 1972 book, *Dr. Atkin's Diet Revolution.* Food pyramids and many other diets followed.

Three recent books are reviewed here that may have a major impact in how we can use nutrition to combat the burden of disease. The lack of nutrition education in medicine is well known. Emerging information from nutrition science calls on medicine to heed the admonition of Hippocrates.

William Davis is a preventive cardiologist in Milwaukee and in his practice promotes a wheat-free diet to lose weight and restore health. The book is well referenced and stays focused on two areas where wheat causes health problems. First he argues that modern engineered wheat with its 42 chromosomes is much different from the 14 chromosome einkorn wheat man began to eat 10,000 years ago and until the last century. Modern wheat is energy dense with the highly glycemic amylopectin A causing blood sugars to rise rapidly and remain high, even more so than many other sweets. The resulting rise in insulin levels causes the deposition of fat, especially central fat.

The second problem with modern wheat is the protein complex known as gluten. Gluten is actually a variety of proteins unique to wheat, barley and rye. Gliadin and glutenin are the two main proteins in gluten and we measure antibodies to these to test for gluten sensitivity. Inflammatory reactions to gluten are common and Davis argues that this is likely a basis for most auto-immune diseases such as inflammatory arthritis and hypothyroidism. Direct inflammatory reactions to gluten may play a leading role in esophageal reflux, irritable bowel disease, acne and rosacea. In *Wheat Belly*, most chapters are focused on the impact of wheat on different organ systems. The evidence here is suggestive and the references are given, and much work needs to be done to nail down what is true.

In *Grain Brain*, David Perlmutter, a neurologist in Naples, FL with a graduate degree in nutrition, argues that wheat and other high glycemic sugars are the basis of many neurodegenerative diseases such as multiple sclerosis, Parkinson disease and Alzheimer's dementia. He argues that the inflammatory nature of gluten and the toxicity of hyperglycemia damage the nervous system.

T. Colin Campbell is a highly respected nutrition scientist originally from Virginia Tech and then Cornell most famous for a large epidemiologic study in Asia called *The China Study* (BenBella Books, 2005). Campbell is well published in scientific journals but went public to get his information better known. He argues for a whole food plant based diet and that animal proteins correlate with many cancers. Casein, the protein in cow's milk, seems to be the worst especially correlating with breast and prostate cancer.

Campbell is a champion of many vegans and Bill Clinton has become an advocate. In *Whole*, Campbell and Jacobson reiterate the data from *The China Study* and argue why reductionist science alone cannot give the answers we need in nutrition. He uses the example of the synergy in an apple when eaten whole gives far more anti-oxidant activity than any of its known ingredients individually. His argument against taking supplements that confuse the body and lack the synergy of whole foods is especially powerful.

Taken together, these three books provide important information about nutrition. We are what we eat and medicine continues to lack sufficient education in food science.

Personally I have benefitted from these books as have my patients. Despite being a marathon runner, for 15 years I had a body mass index of 26 and a 36-inch waist (I had a 32-inch waist my first 15 years of adult life, and a 34-inch waist the second 15 years). I enjoyed bread and whole grain cereals. Four months after giving up wheat my waist became 32 inches and I lost 20 pounds with a body mass index of 21. Interestingly, the emerging rosacea on my nose went away. My patients that become wheat free and do not replace wheat with other starches report similar weight loss and health benefits. And, I am now drinking almond milk.

I used my new knowledge of the role of carbohydrates in obesity and the health problems caused by gluten to summarize recent research articles for the publication *Internal Medicine Alert*. These articles are reprinted here and the references are at the end of the book.

The Obesity Epidemic and How We Got Wrong

Internal Medicine Alert
June 29, 2014

Synopsis: There are now 2.1 billion overweight and obese people in the world, up from 857 million people in 1980. The epidemic is global and the U.S. leads the increase among developed countries. This rise coincided with many factors including the development of low fat foods, thinking that saturated fat was the main dietary problem. Recent evidence suggests that the ingestion of high glycemic carbohydrates is the main problem with overweight and obesity and intake of these products increased after the introduction of low fat foods. Grain based starches have among the highest glycemic index even exceeding that of the table sugar.

Source: Ng M, Fleming T, Robinson M, et al. Global, regional, and national prevalence of overweight and obesity in children and adults during 1980-2013: A systematic analysis for the Global Burden of Disease Study 2013. The Lancet. 2014; 10.1016/S0140-6736 (14)60460-8. [Epub ahead of print].

The numbers are startling. Worldwide the rates of overweight and obesity have soared in the last 33 years according to the Global Burden of Disease Study 2013, funded by the Bill and Melinda Gates Foundation in cooperation with the World Health Organization. Over half of the obese people live in 10 countries: The USA, China, India, Russia, Brazil, Mexico, Egypt, Germany,

Pakistan and Indonesia, showing that obesity is no longer tied to culture or socioeconomic status. There has been a 28% increase overweight and obesity in adults and a 47% increase in children. This robust study looks at both gender and age with respect to rates of overweight and obesity among different countries.

Commentary

Many factors converge to cause overweight and obesity. Most populations have become more sedentary, with increased urbanization. More people eat away from home than previously, especially at "fast food" restaurants. Interestingly, the rise in overweight and obesity starting in the 1980s coincided with the recognition that elevated blood cholesterol is a cardiac risk factor and the development of a low fat food industry.

Thinking that fats, especially saturated fats, are a risk factor for heart disease is logical but is not borne out by the data.[1,2] In his popular book, *Grain Brain*, neurologist and nutritionist David Perlmutter, lays out the benefits of saturated fats, especially on the neurologic system, and describes the dangers of elevated blood sugar coming from ingesting high glycemic carbohydrates.[3]

Body fat, especially around the trunk, is associated with hyperlipidemia and the other components of the metabolic syndrome, raising cardiovascular risk. The foods that are most associated with increasing body fat are the high glycemic carbohydrates. Cardiologist William Davis lays out this data well in his popular book, *Wheat Belly*.[4]

The glycemic index of foods is a nutritional measure of how much the blood sugar rises in the 90 to 120 minutes after a food is consumed. This measure was developed in a study at the University of Toronto published in 1981.[5] Pure glucose has a glycemic index of 100. Interestingly grain based starches have a higher glycemic index than table sugar.[6] Whole grain bread has a glycemic index of 72, white bread 68, wheat cereal 67 and table sugar 59.[4-6]

High glycemic foods trigger rapid insulin release and ultimately the conversion and storage of body fat in persons who are not working or exercising vigorously. High glycemic carbohydrates also drive hunger as rising and falling blood sugars trigger the desire to eat. Replacing fat with carbohydrates, especially grain based foods, has coincided with an increase in calories consumed.[7]

Thirty years of discouraging saturated fats and promoting whole grains has been misguided. It is not just about calories in and calories out. The hormonal responses to the calories we eat play a major role in how much we eat and what happens in our body. The problem is excess body fat, especially in the trunk. The nutritional approach to curbing overweight and obesity is to reduce the foods that contribute most to appetite and body fat, and those are the high glycemic carbohydrates, especially grain based foods.

Does Gluten Cause Health Problems in Patients Without Celiac Disease?

Internal Medicine Alert
August 29, 2014

Synopsis: Gluten is a protein complex that may be inflammatory to humans and is increasingly recognized as a possible cause of numerous health problems such as irritable bowel syndrome, fibromyalgia, skin conditions, allergies, auto-immune arthritis and neurodegenerative conditions.

Source: Volta U, Bardella MT, Calabro A, Troncone R, Corazza GR, et al. An Italian prospective multicenter survey on patients suspected of having non-celiac gluten sensitivity. BMC Med. 2014;12:85.

These Italian investigators enlisted 38 clinical sites (27 adult gastroenterology, 5 internal medicine, 4 pediatrics and 2 allergy) to distribute a questionnaire aimed at identifying patients with health problems possibly associated with non-celiac gluten sensitivity. 486 patients were identified over a one year period, most were female and the mean age was 38 years.

The clinical symptoms associated with gluten were a variety of gastrointestinal complaints: abdominal pain, bloating, diarrhea and/or constipation, nausea, epigastric pain, GERD and aphthous stomatitis. Other complaints included fatigue, fibromyalgia, headache, joint and muscle pain, "foggy mind", dermatitis or skin rash, depression and anxiety. The most frequent diagnoses in these patients were irritable bowel syndrome (47%), food intolerance (35%) and IgE mediated allergy (22%). The time lag between ingestion of gluten and the symptoms varied from a few hours to one day. Diagnostic tests for celiac disease were negative in these patients and those who underwent duodenal biopsy showed normal intestinal mucosa.

The authors conclude that non-celiac gluten sensitivity appears to be associated with a large number of health problems.

Commentary

Non-celiac gluten sensitivity is still medically undefined, but is emerging as a possible probable cause of multiple health problems. Dr. William Davis brought this to light with his 2011 book *Wheat Belly.*[1] Since then there have been multiple reports of remission of conditions with the elimination of gluten, and their relapse when gluten is ingested.[2-7] This area remains controversial and is criticized by many leading food science centers.

Gluten is not a distinct chemical, but a protein complex consisting of two types of proteins, gliadins and glutenins. Measurement of antibodies to these proteins is used to diagnose celiac disease. Patients with non-gluten sensitivity usually have negative tests for celiac so the diagnosis requires food elimination and clinical judgment. Like other nutritional conditions, using the food, withdrawing it and using it again has diagnostic validity.

William Davis describes in detail how modern wheat is much different than the original wheat used before 1950.[1] Through hybridization, wheat has become much more energy dense with 42 chromosomes compared with the 14 chromosomes of ancient einkorn wheat.

The number of clinical conditions associated with gluten ingestion is staggering. The strongest evidence seems to be with GI distress, skin conditions (my rosacea went away when I stopped gluten and comes back if I ingest it), allergies and fibromyalgia. If these associations are borne out by controlled studies, the burden of disease could be markedly reduced. It is not clear how much of the population is gluten sensitive. The Italian study questionnaire was positive for a small percentage of patients, similar to the prevalence of celiac disease (around 2%). However the real incidence is likely much higher. The association of chronic gluten ingestion and neurodegenerative conditions such as multiple sclerosis, Parkinson's disease and other tremor, and even Alzheimer's disease is alarming.[8] These are described briefly by William Davis[1] and in more detail by neurologist Dr. David Perlmutter in his book, *Grain Brain*.[9]

As we learn more about the power of nutrition and the intestinal microbiome, a new area of clinical medicine is opening up. NIH does not have an institute solely devoted to nutritional research, something that nutrition experts regret.[10] I am finding that the longer I am in medicine, the more I follow the words of Hippocrates, "Let food be thy medicine and medicine be thy food".

Wheat Causes Intestinal Immune Activation in Some People Without Celiac Disease

Internal Medicine Alert
August 3, 2016

Synopsis: Some people without celiac disease may exhibit wheat sensitivity with demonstrated intestinal epithelial cell damage.

Source: Uhde M, Ajamian M, Caio G, et al. Intestinal cell damage and systemic immune activation in individuals reporting sensitivity to wheat in the absence of coeliac disease. Gut. 2016;0:1-8, doi:10.1136/gutnl-2016-311964. Published online July 25, 2016.

A team at Columbia University studied 80 individuals who reported on a standardized questionnaire sensitivity to wheat, rye or barley. These subjects were compared with 40 individuals with celiac disease and 40 healthy individuals with no symptoms. Those with non-celiac wheat sensitivity (NCWS) experienced intestinal symptoms (bloating, abdominal pain, diarrhea, epigastric pain and nausea) and extraintestinal symptoms (fatigue, headache, anxiety, memory and cognitive disturbances, and numbness of the arms or legs). These symptoms improved or disappeared when wheat, rye and barley were removed for 6 months. The symptoms recurred when these foods were re-introduced for up to 1 month.

Serum samples and intestinal biopsies were performed on all the study subjects and controls. Those with NCWS did not have the IgA antibodies or TG2 autoantibodies specific for celiac disease. They also did not have the intestinal histologic findings specific for celiac disease. Those with NCWS did show changes in the serum and intestinal epithelium not seen in the healthy controls. These findings include increased levels of soluble CD14 and lipopolysaccharide-binding protein indicating systemic immune activation. NCWS subjects also showed increased levels of fatty acid-binding protein 2 suggesting compromised intestinal barrier integrity. The intestinal biopsies of subjects with NCWS showed epithelial cell damage not seen in healthy controls and different from the changes seen in celiac disease. These abnormalities largely resolved during the 6 months off the offending foods.

Commentary

This study provides further biologic evidence for the "leaky gut" changes postulated in people consuming the gluten containing foods of wheat, rye and barley. These authors chose to use wheat and related grains as the culprits since other proteins may be involved beyond the gluten complex of gliadins and glutamines. The prevalence of NCWS is unknown, and it is not clear if most people complaining of "gluten sensitivity" have any of these changes.

The range of intestinal and extraintestinal symptoms experienced by these subjects is impressive, including their resolution after removal of the offending foods. These results match with my practice experience. I routinely recommend the removal of wheat, rye and barley from all patients with gastroesophageal reflux (GERD) and irritable bowel syndrome, with clinical improvement or resolution of symptoms in most patients. I am gratified to get many patients off their PPI or H2 blocking medications. I also find that many patients with chronic fatigue and fibromyalgia symptoms improve or recover with elimination of these foods. The full list of symptoms and diagnoses associated with inflammatory grains is quite long.

This study did not address the association of inflammatory grains with a variety of auto-immune diseases. This area and the role of the gut microbiome have been explored in other reports.[1-6]

The specific biologic results shown in this controlled study should help us recognize the importance of understanding how inflammatory grains may be harming our patients. The time is now to use an elimination diet with many of our patients.

My first year on this new nutrition had me about 90% compliant and feeling much healthier. I felt like I had turned back the clock by a decade and my running times demonstrated that. My half marathon times had been over 2 hours from my early 50s to age 63 and now were back under 2 hours. My marathon times improved by 20 minutes.

I continued to read books on the new nutrition and it was clear I should go 100% into low carbohydrate living and that story is covered next.

PART 4: THE SCIENCE OF LOW CARBOHYDRATE LIVING AND PERFORMANCE

Reading and learning more about healthy nutrition intensified my commitment to a healthy diet of whole foods and being free of grains and low carbohydrate intake daily. This may sound difficult or complicated but it is not. I just follow the simple rules of not eating grains, avoiding cow's milk (except for some half and half in coffee), and limiting carbohydrates. The amount of foods available is abundant and no dieting such as calorie counting is involved. By age 65 my waist was still the 32 inches I enjoyed as a young man in my 20s. That felt great and my running and hiking required much less effort. The next phase of my journey took me deeper into the science.

Jeff Volek is an academic nutrition scientist at The Ohio State University. He is an RD (Registered Dietician) and has a PhD in nutrition. Stephen Phinney is a physician with a PhD in nutrition and recently retired from the University of California, Davis. Together they have written two recent and very important books, *The Art and Science of*

Low Carbohydrate Living (2011) and *The Art and Science of Low Carbohydrate Performance* (2012). They provide the science behind the work started by Robert Atkins in the 1960s.

The Robert Atkins story is most interesting. It all began with a small study done at the University of Wisconsin and published in the Journal of the American Medical Association (JAMA) in 1963. After reading the two books by Volek and Phinney, I went back and read the 1972 book, *Dr. Atkin's Diet Revolution.* I was amazed by how much of the science of low carbohydrate nutrition was there. Dr. Atkins improved his description of his diet in his 1992 and subsequent editions of *Dr. Atkins New Diet Revolution.*

I wrote an article about the life and courage of Robert Atkins, and could not find a journal willing to publish it. So here it is:

Profile in Courage – Robert Atkins

That which seems the height of absurdity in one generation often becomes the height of wisdom in another.
John Stuart Mill[1]

Like many physicians educated in the 1970s and for three decades after, I thought Robert Atkins was a kook. As the data accumulated that high cholesterol was a major risk factor for heart disease, and that eating saturated fat most likely contributed to this problem, how dare a physician recommend a diet high in saturated fat and low in the whole grains that provided fiber and other nutrients.

Whatever weight loss that happened on an Atkins diet must be water and temporary, and the diet must be unhealthy.

Recent research is proving Atkins was largely correct. Carbohydrates are the main driver of excess body fat and the changes in the lipids that increase cardiovascular risk.[2-7] Carbohydrates drive hunger by raising insulin levels and causing wide variations in blood sugar. Replacing fat with carbohydrates, especially grain based foods, has coincided with an increase in calories consumed.[6]

Eating saturated fat increases satiety and provides sustained energy, increases lean body mass and ultimately results in lower body fat.[4,5] Body fat, especially in the trunk, is the primary lesion of the metabolic syndrome risk factors and is increased through high carbohydrate intake.[5,7]

The background of Robert Atkins is both ordinary and impressive. He was born in Columbus, Ohio in 1930 and at the age of 12 the family moved to Dayton. They owned several restaurants. His undergraduate degree was from the University of Michigan. He attended Cornell University Medical College (now Weill Cornell Medical College). After an internship at Strong Hospital in Rochester, NY, he completed his internal medicine residency and fellowship in cardiology at Columbia University. He opened a medical practice in the Upper East Side of Manhattan in 1959.[8]

The Atkins diet did not originate with him. In 1963, at age 33, Dr. Atkins was morbidly obese at 224 lbs. and saw a triple chin in the mirror. He read an article in JAMA that advocated a low carbohydrate diet and marked increase in both protein and fat.[9] Atkins found rapid success on this eating plan and began to advocate it for his patients, with equal success. Atkins appeared on The Tonight Show in 1965 and Vogue magazine published his eating plan in 1970 and his diet was originally known as "the Vogue Diet".[8]

Robert Atkins published his groundbreaking book, *Dr. Atkins' Diet Revolution*, in 1972 just as the low fat recommendations were being established and a low fat food industry developed.[10] Ironically, the American Medical Association Council on Nutrition publishing in JAMA condemned the diet that Atkins had developed from a JAMA article 10 years earlier.[11] Americans bought into the low fat food paradigm and Atkins was to be dismissed by the scientific community for decades up to his accidental death from head trauma in 2003.

Did Atkins promote the reckless consumption of unhealthy foods? No. I combed his 1972 book for excessive and unhealthy fats. He refers to his diet as steak plus salad plus. While he called for zero carbohydrates, he promoted vegetables and some fruits. What he meant was zero consumption of sugars and refined starches.[10] Ahead of his time, Atkins referred to type 2 diabetes and other hyperglycemia as "carbohydrate intolerance", a term that is being promoted today.[5] In 1972 he described insulin resistance and how high blood sugars result in increased fat deposition.[10]

I was in medical school when his first book came out and was taught that the presence of ketones in the blood or urine meant starvation or acidosis. Having ketones in the blood and urine reflects the burning of fat, the best source of sustained energy. Atkins promoted a ketogenic diet to lose weight, something that is being highly recommended by nutrition scientists today, even for high performance athletes.[13]

Atkins' 1992 book and two subsequent editions up to 2002 were equally popular and showed his diet was not a fad.[14] The updates were an embrace of "controlled" carbohydrate eating with more vegetables and some fruits. He advocated the use of the glycemic index of carbohydrates developed at the University of Toronto in 1981.[15] Atkins actively promoted the intake of foods we consider "superfoods" today: spinach, broccoli, kale and berries.

There is room for criticism in the work of Robert Atkins. Despite establishing a multimillion dollar operation, he failed to do research in any meaningful way. He started to promote supplements without an evidence base, and had the conflict of starting his own company that sold nutraceuticals. It became apparent that the later editions of his "Diet Revolution" books were written by a committee with variable quality and making the diet approach more complicated.

These problems and Atkins death in 2003 opened the door for other low carbohydrate diet programs. Another cardiologist, Arthur Agatston, brought forward the widely successful South Beach Diet in 2003.[16] Agatston started work in weight loss in the 1990s and altered the Atkins approach by further differentiating "good carbs" from "bad carbs" based on the glycemic index and "good fats" from "bad fats" based on promoting unsaturated fats over saturated fats. Agatston promoted the South Beach Diet as more "heart healthy" than the Atkins Diet. Today's exoneration of saturated fats calls into question whether the

Atkins' Diet was actually less heart healthy than the South Beach Diet.

Currently low carbohydrate diets are gaining wide favor. Another cardiologist, William Davis, simplified the approach in his book *Wheat Belly* calling for the elimination of all flour based foods, especially wheat that also has the inflammatory protein complex gluten.[7] I lost 20 pounds in 4 months and optimized my weight, body fat, blood sugar and lipids using this simple approach, and it has worked very well with my patients. The current Paleo Diet accomplishes the same goal by eliminating the high glycemic flour based and processed foods.[17,18]

Three nutrition scientists, two are physicians at major academic centers, provide a large body of research in favor of the Atkins diet, using the themes of "the right carbs in the right amounts", "the power of protein", and "meet your new friend: fat".[19] A recent randomized controlled trial of low carbohydrate versus low fat nutrition expanded the data in favor of low carb by showing that eating more fat and less carbs not only reduces body fat, but also reduces inflammatory markers including small LDL particle size, and increases lean body mass. Eating more carbohydrates and less fat causes the opposite unhealthy effects.[2]

Walter Willett of the Harvard School of Public Health has been vocal that fat is not the problem and evidence does not support the recommendation to eat less saturated fat, and that excess carbohydrates are to blame for obesity, diabetes and other metabolic diseases.[20,21] With a similar message, David Perlmutter is lecturing widely after his 2013 book *Grain Brain*.[22] Mark Hyman of *The Daniel Plan* has been hired by the Cleveland Clinic to lead a Functional Medicine Institute.[23,24]

Many nutrition questions remain. What about cancer? If cardiovascular disease is reduced by a low carbohydrate diet, premature death from cancer and other diseases likely affected by nutrition may increase. The generous animal protein advocated by Atkins may still be unhealthy particularly as animals are fed from grain rather than grass. Those advocating a whole food plant based diet have the strongest data to support cancer prevention.[25,26] The power of nutrition is much greater than given credit in medical education and medical research. May the debates begin between the vegan and Paleo diets through further study.

While Atkins made millions from his books, he was ostracized from his profession. For decades his work came up against the recommendations of scientific authorities, government bodies and organizations such as the American Heart Association (AHA). Now that low carbohydrate eating is rapidly gaining favor, Atkins' name still remains tarnished. It is politically correct to say that you are recommending a "modified" Atkins diet. It is time we gave Robert Atkins the respect he deserves for being a pioneer in combating overweight and obesity.

Wanting to contribute to the literature on low carbohydrate nutrition I reworked the Atkins article and the following was published in *The San Diego Physician* in 2015. Some redundancy is in what follows here.

Overweight and Obesity – It's the Carbohydrates

The awareness that a low carbohydrate diet rich in protein and saturated fat resulted in a lower body weight has a long history. In 1927 nutritionist Gayelord Hauser came to Hollywood and helped Greta Garbo, Marlene Dietrich and other stars stay lean by avoiding sugars and foods made with flour. Hauser published 19 books between 1930 and 1963 with the most famous being *Look Younger, Live Longer* (1950).[1]

In 1963 the Journal of the American Medical Association (JAMA) published an article from the University of Wisconsin on a novel low carbohydrate diet that achieved rapid weight loss.[2] A young obese Manhattan cardiologist named Robert Atkins read the article and tried the diet. He lost his excess weight rapidly and began using it with patients with great success. Atkins appeared on The Tonight Show in 1965 and Vogue magazine did a story on the diet and it became known as the "Vogue diet" in 1970.[3] In 1972 Atkins published his first "Diet Revolution" book and the very low carbohydrate diet rich in fats and protein become known as the Atkins diet.[4] Other popular diets followed calling themselves a "modified Atkins", such as The South Beach Diet in 2003.[5]

Meanwhile, in the 1970s mainstream medicine realized that lipids were an important risk factor for cardiovascular disease, the top killer in the industrialized world. By a leap of faith and rational thinking more than good science, the mainstream nutrition and medical community blamed dietary saturated fat for causing high cholesterol and launched new recommended diet programs of less fat and more carbohydrates, especially complex carbohydrates such as "healthy whole grains". Starting in 1980, the overweight and obesity epidemic took off with exponential rises in these conditions over the next three decades.

Recent research is showing that the low carbohydrate diet is largely correct for maintaining a healthy weight.[6-10] Carbohydrates are the main driver of excess body fat by causing fluctuations in blood sugar that increase appetite. Increasing blood sugar causes insulin secretion that drives sugar into cells. What is not burned for energy or stored in the muscles and liver becomes stored fat through lipogenesis. Body fat is hormonally active and causes the four problems of the metabolic syndrome: dyslipidemia, elevated blood sugar, elevated blood pressure and overweight/obesity. There is a genetic contribution to all this but the ill effects of carbohydrate intake beyond our energy needs are universal. Excess sugar converted into fat storage reduces LDL particle size and stimulates inflammatory changes in blood vessels leading to atherosclerosis.[6] Replacing fat with carbohydrates, especially grain based foods, has coincided with an increase in calories consumed.[9,10] Carbohydrates are best obtained from vegetables and whole fruits. Eating more saturated fat and protein reduces hunger and results in fewer calories consumed, the key to the success of low carbohydrate diets.

Two academic nutrition scientists, Jeff Volek, PhD, RD, and Stephen Phinney, MD, PhD, have gathered the science around the low carbohydrate diet in their book for professionals, *The Art and Science of Low Carbohydrate Living*.[9] Their work and others have vindicated the approach taken by Robert Atkins that saturated fat should be a mainstay of a healthy diet. Eating saturated fat from natural sources such as tree nuts, avocados, eggs, meat and fish reduces hunger and overall calorie intake resulting in lower body fat.

Volek and Phinney have also triggered a trend among high performance endurance athletes to move away from carbohydrate loading and sweetened energy drinks. They show that a ketogenic diet of steady fat burning will improve performance over burning a temporary supply of carbohydrates.[11] Humans are not like hybrid cars readily able to convert from one energy source to another, in our case from carbohydrate to fat burning. If athletes depend on carbs for energy, there is a drop in energy and muscle cramps when they run out. No more pasta before events, eat the steak! Drink water rather than sweet energy drinks and gels and get necessary salt, fat and protein during long events such as a marathons and ultramarathons, triathlons, bicycle races and hiking.

Men's professional tennis is a grueling sport especially in major events that can go to 5 sets and over 4 hours. Of the leading male tennis professionals, Novak Djokovic follows a very low carbohydrate diet and relies on fat burning during performances.[12] Interestingly in the 2015 Australian Open, the semi-final had Djokovic facing defending champion Stan Wawrinka in a match that went 5 sets. The score in the final set was Djokovic 6-0. In the final Djokovic faced Brad Murray in a 4 set match. The score in the final set was Djokovic 6-0. What role did diet play in this success with endurance?

The dominant cause and solution to the overweight and obesity epidemic remains hidden in plain sight – it's the carbohydrates. The food industry flourishes on selling foods made with flour and sugar. These food commodities are the easiest to package and store, and hence result in greater profits. The food industry also funds major health organizations, nutritional research institutes and federal agencies that provide dietary recommendations, resulting in much inertia to change.[13,14]

Countering the status quo of boxes of high carbohydrate foods lining our supermarket aisles is a growing worldwide realization that eating the food that nature has provided for millions of years is better for us than the more recent breads and processed foods. The Paleo Diet was introduced in 1975 and is becoming a new fashion whether people understand the nutrition behind it or not.[15,16] French physician Pierre Dukan has been promoting a low carbohydrate diet for over 30 years and the Dukan Diet is increasingly popular in Great Britain and France.[17]

Walter Willett of the Harvard School of Public Health has been vocal that fat is not the problem and evidence does not support the recommendation against eating less saturated fat, and that excess carbohydrates are to blame for obesity, diabetes and other metabolic diseases.[20,21] A growing number of physician innovators are using the evidence about carbohydrates to educate the public, including William Davis,[12,18] David Perlmutter[19] and Mark Hyman, nutrition advisor to Bill Clinton and recently hired by the Cleveland Clinic to lead a new Functional Medicine Institute.[20]

Paradigm changes in science and medicine happen slowly. Thomas Kuhn observed that "normal science" is predicated on the assumption that the scientific community knows what the world is like, and scientists take great pains to defend those assumptions. Scientists tend to ignore research findings that might threaten the existing paradigm and trigger the development of new and competing beliefs. Changing a scientific paradigm only happens through discovery brought on by repeated encounters with anomaly.[21] The paradigm around what is a healthy diet is changing from low fat to a low carbohydrate diet rich in natural fats and proteins.

Low carbohydrate nutrition and athletic performance is a revolutionary development and demonstrates that carbohydrate loading and carbohydrate energy drinks and gels are a mistake for athletes needing to perform for hours. As Volek and Phinney describe, with the data to support it, we can only store limited carbohydrate energy. On the other hand, even with a very low body fat, we store much more fat energy, a difference of 2000 calories of carbohydrate energy compared with 80,000 calories of fat energy. If we load up with carbohydrates, we will preferentially burn that until it is depleted. We are not as efficient as hybrid cars able to readily switch from one energy source to another. When we deplete our carbohydrates we get muscle cramps and feel dizzy.

If we follow a low carbohydrate diet, such as not more than 50 grams of carbohydrate daily from natural foods, we become a fat burner. This transition in our body takes a few months to develop. Once it happens, we can perform for many hours with a stable blood sugar and no drop in energy. We become ketogenic (ketones are the breakdown products of fat) and use our tremendous stores of fat energy as our fuel from the beginning.

As I write this, the U.S. Open tennis tournament is underway and despite fine weather, large numbers of players are cramping up and withdrawing from their matches. The high carbohydrate snacks cannot keep them going. Meanwhile Novak Djokovic just keeps going.

I experienced this effect in my marathon running, and follow a low carbohydrate diet. With no carbohydrate loading and avoiding carbs at the rest stops, instead having some fat and protein such as from dark chocolate and nuts, and drinking only water, I just keep going. I am now able to sprint over the finish line with better times.

As I became fully devoted to low carbohydrate eating, I enjoy the health benefits of a constant clear headedness. I also believe that I have reduced my risks of the chronic diseases that plague us as we age, hopefully avoiding the Parkinson's disease of my father. My knowledge journey was far from over as I describe in the final part of this book.

PART 5: TOTAL HEALTH IN BODY AND MIND

"No disease that can be treated by diet should be treated with any other means".
Maimonides

I started this journey to low carbohydrate nutrition three years before this writing by reading William Davis, a cardiologist who reversed his type 2 diabetes and excess body fat by giving up all wheat products, and David Perlmutter, the neurologist described earlier. After these two physicians published their original works, they went on social media and learned from the wisdom of the crowds of people who embrace this nutrition revolution. They also became leaders in a new medical field called functional medicine. Functional medicine seeks to find the root causes of disease and repair that rather than simply treat disease with drugs and procedures.

The excess carbohydrates causing overweight and obesity is straightforward. Carbohydrates create an unstable blood sugar and we become hungry when our blood sugar is falling. The high carbohydrate American diet results in our eating about 30% more calories that we would if we consumed more fats from natural sources (William Davis, *Wheat Belly*).

The impact of the inflammatory proteins of grains on our health is much more complex. This is explored in the second book by William Davis, *Wheat Belly Total Health* (2014). Prolamin proteins such as the gluten complex cause a leaky gut phenomenon where proteins from the intestine never meant for our bloodstream get in and cause an inflammatory immune reaction. In some people with repeated exposure to these proteins an auto-immune condition develops with our own antibodies attacking different organs of our body. The entire range of auto-immune diseases, hypothyroidism, rheumatoid and other inflammatory arthritis conditions, skin diseases such as acne, rosacea and psoriasis, neurological diseases such as multiple sclerosis, may be caused by our nutrition. Most of these diseases are unique to humans and are not found in the animal kingdom eating food from natural sources. The burden of diseases that appear to be caused by this malnutrition is staggering.

David Perlmutter in his second book, *Brain Maker* (2015) brings the early knowledge of the intestinal microbiome into the picture. We have about 100 trillion bacteria in and on our body, 10 times the number of cells, and most of these bacteria are in our gut. They determine our health in ways previously unimagined. These bacteria are completely determined by what we eat, and they change accordingly. A healthy whole food diet results in a healthy microbiome and unhealthy eating, especially inflammatory proteins, causes an unhealthy microbiome and the gut phenomenon described above. Our intestinal bacteria have a direct connection to the health of our brains and an unhealthy microbiome through malnutrition may be the underlying cause of neurodegeneration culminating in Alzheimer's dementia.

I have written book reviews of both of these works published in *Family Medicine* and presented here:

Wheat Belly Total Health

William Davis, MD
New York: Rodale, 2014

In his 2011 book, *Wheat Belly,* William Davis presented a new perspective on low carbohydrate nutrition.[1] He argued that the high glycemic index and high glycemic load of grains, especially wheat, were primary drivers of overweight, obesity and type 2 diabetes. The so called "healthy whole wheat" increased hunger though elevated blood sugars and the pouring out of insulin causing people to eat about 30% more calories. In addition, he argued that the inflammatory protein complex gluten in wheat, barley and rye is associated with a large burden of disease in multiple organ systems.

William Davis is a cardiologist practicing near Milwaukee. As he describes in his follow-up book, *Wheat Belly Total Health*, he was obese, had type 2 diabetes and dyslipidemia with an HDL cholesterol of 27. All of this reversed when he gave up eating grains.

After *Wheat Belly,* Davis used social media to create a dialogue on his website, wheatbellyblog.com and on Facebook. He became further educated by the "wisdom of the crowd" and *Wheat Belly Total Health* is the result. It is much denser delving into the principles and practice of functional medicine and their approach to nutrition.[2] All grains become the target and Davis argues that non-gluten seeds of grasses such as oats, corn and rice are as inflammatory to the human body as gluten.

Wheat Belly Total Health is divided into three parts: No Grain is a Good Grain, Living Grainlessly, and Be a Grainless Overachiever. The clear organization stops there as the text becomes scattered. Problems with the GI tract, nervous system and thyroid are presented multiple times with varying degrees of detail. While *Wheat Belly Total Health* has more nutritional depth than *Wheat Belly,* its lack of coherency makes it a more frustrating read, especially for patients lacking a background in nutrition and inflammatory health problems.

Low carbohydrate and anti-inflammatory nutrition are trends that have mounting scientific evidence, and should be part of the teaching of medical students, residents and physicians in practice. There is now well documented high quality evidence that a low carbohydrate diet is superior to the low fat diet the American Heart Association has recommended for decades.[3] Evidence for the inflammatory effects of gluten in non-celiac patients has accumulated in observational studies from around the world.[4,5]

Like other popular books promoting a certain nutrition, Davis exaggerates the evidence. From the beginning of the book, he boasts from a one-sided perspective. There is no expression of humility and little expression of a need for more evidence. Evidence of benefit from grain based fiber is dismissed outright. Despite these limitations the book is important and worth recommending to learners and patients. I recommend reading *Wheat Belly* first as an introduction and then *Wheat Belly Total Health* for a deeper dive into grain free nutrition.

The most valuable parts of *Wheat Belly Total Health* are the explanations of why some people do not lose weight with the elimination of grains. There is a good explanation of thyroid function, especially the conversion of the storage hormone T4 into the active hormone T3 that may be blocked by chronic ingestion of grains. I am now ordering more Free T3 tests with TSH in overweight and obese patients. When the Free T3 is low, an addition of T3 in the treatment may result in rapid weight loss. Deficiencies of iodine and vitamin D are also discussed in detail.

There is a large inconvenient truth emerging in the nutrition science that foods many Americans enjoy, bread, cookies, cakes, bagels, and tortillas, are unhealthy. Grains have been hybridized to become much more energy dense than the original forms found in nature. The high glycemic consequences are seen in an overweight and obese society. Coupled with the burden of disease postulated from inflammatory foods, there is much to be said for going grain free. William Davis, along with neurologist David Perlmutter[6,7] and family physician Mark Hyman,[8] are committed physician authors grounded in functional medicine and well worth making part of the educational dialogue of nutrition science.

Brain Maker

David Perlmutter, MD with Kristin Loberg
New York: Little, Brown and Co. 2015

You are what you feed your gut microbiome. That is the central message of David Perlmutter's second book on nutrition and the health of the brain. In his first book *Grain Brain* (Little, Brown and Co. 2013), Perlmutter discussed how elevated blood sugar from grains and sweets combined with the inflammatory proteins of grains to cause much of the neurodegenerative conditions afflicting humans including Alzheimer's disease. In *Brain Maker* Perlmutter brings forth the emerging science on the gut microbiome and how it affects the brain and our overall health.

This is an important book that describes scientifically, with some hyperbole, a new frontier in medicine. The NIH started the Human Microbiome Project in 2008 and what is coming out of this is a whole new organ system affecting human health.[1] While the 100 trillion organisms are segregated in the gut, orifices and the skin, they chemically interact throughout the body. The gut microbiome develops after birth and is completely dependent on what we eat.

Brain Maker is divided into three parts. Part 1 describes the gut microbiome and its impact on health and disease. Whether we are born sterile is not completely known, there may be *in utero* microbiome development, but for the most part our gut microbiome is initiated at birth through the vaginal birth canal. Perlmutter describes the risks involved with Cesarean birth and describes how gauze with vaginal fluids may be applied to a baby's mouth. Breastfeeding is ideal for getting the gut microbiome off to a healthy start.

Part 2 describes what goes wrong. Gluten and fructose, abundant in our common foods, lead to inflammation in the body by negatively impacting the gut microbiome. The proteins of grains, specifically the gluten protein complex, and high fructose corn syrup in sweets, combine to cause inflammatory reactions starting in the gut. The biology of "leaky gut" is described in common language for a public audience but also with solid scientific detail. The leakage of inflammatory proteins from the gut into the bloodstream and their effect on mitochondria set the stage for auto-immune disease.

The information that our gut microbiome affects our mood and may contribute to anxiety and depression is becoming well known.[2] Perlmutter goes much further and makes an impressive case that an unhealthy gut microbiome is the likely cause of Autism Spectrum Disorders. Case reports are included about the reversal of symptoms in Autism and Tourette syndrome that may be accomplished through probiotic enemas and fecal transplantation.

In Part 3 Perlmutter gives his recommendations for developing and maintaining a healthy gut microbiome. He emphasizes fermented foods such as yogurt, kefir and pickled foods as the stars of a good diet. He emphasizes a low carbohydrate, high-quality fat diet and lists the "brain maker foods". He recommends some supplements including probiotics, especially when taking an antibiotic, and DHA, turmeric, coconut oil, alpha-lipoic acid, and vitamin D. Overall Perlmutter does not push supplements as much as he did in *Grain Brain*.

Many people reading this book will feel that Perlmutter goes way too far in his statements and recommendations, and they may be right, but there is new knowledge and therapeutic breakthroughs that will further develop in this new area of science and medicine.

In summary, *Brain Maker* is worth reading and recommending to learners and patients, with some caveats. Perlmutter is daring and the full truth about what he presents will take time but the reader will be impressed with the overall message. I tell patients to focus on Part 3 of the book and bring me their questions. The emergence of knowledge about our gut microbiome makes what we eat even more important to our health. The old expression "you are what you eat" is being modified to include an important intermediary, the gut microbiome.

Research on the importance of the gut microbiome is exploding and I explored the connection between the gut microbiome and the brain further with this article in *Internal Medicine Alert*:

You Are What You Feed Your Gut Microbiome

Internal Medicine Alert
August 29, 2015

Synopsis: The human gut microbiome regulates intestinal function and health. There is mounting evidence that the gut microbiome influences the immune system and the central and peripheral nervous systems. This article reviews the bidirectional relationship between the gut microbiome and brain disorders.

Source: Petra AI, Panagiotidou S, Hatziagelaki E, et al. Gut-Microbiota-Brain Axis and its Effect on

Neuropsychiatric Disorders With Suspected Immune Dysfunction. Clin Ther. 2015;37:984-995.

These authors reviewed articles on Medline starting in 1980 for a wide range of neurologic disorders and two systems, the gut-microbiota-brain axis and the hypothalamic-pituitary-adrenal axis. Bidirectional influences exist between the brain and the gut flora that are associated with mood disorders, autism-spectrum disorders, attention-deficit hypersensitivity disorder, multiple sclerosis and obesity. This article joins a growing list of other studies illuminating these relationships.[1-4]

Bacterial dysbiosis, small intestinal bacterial overgrowth, and increased intestinal permeability may produce numerous immunologic effects including central nervous system inflammation. Our mood is affected by these changes. Bacterial proteins cross-react with human antigens to stimulate dysfunctional responses of the immune system that may lead to neurodegenerative disorders.

Communication between the gut and the brain goes both ways. Antibiotics, environmental and infectious agents, intestinal neurotransmitters, sensory vagal fibers, cytokines and essential metabolites all convey information to the central nervous system (CNS) about the intestinal state. The hypothalamic-pituitary-adrenal axis is the CNS regulatory area of satiety, and neuropeptides released from sensory nerve fibers affect the gut microbiota composition directly or through nutrient availability. Such interactions appear to influence the pathogenesis of a number of nervous system disorders, from mood to auto-immune neurodegenerative conditions to obesity.

Commentary

"You are what you eat" is an age old expression highlighting that we are organisms that depend on food for growth and survival. The title even became a popular diet and TV program in the United Kingdom from 2004-2007. With the emphasis in modern medicine on pharmacologic therapies and procedures, the vital importance of nutrition has been downplayed in human health and disease. Many people eat whatever they want and health care does little to intervene. We continue to have debates on what constitutes a healthy diet.

The recent appreciation of the gut microbiome, the 100 trillion organisms that resides within us, has added a new dimension to this expression. These gut bacteria together weigh about 10 pounds and would occupy a half gallon container. They are a new vital organ to the human species. They completely depend on us for sustenance.

The gut microbiome is an important intermediary between what we eat and our health. The gut bacteria get first crack at what we eat and play a vital role in what gets into our bodies and what happens to these nutrients. A healthy gut microbiome is critical for good health and an unhealthy gut microbiome assures that we will not be well.

The science around the gut microbiome is in its infancy. The Human Microbiome Project at the NIH was established in 2008.[5] The emerging knowledge from this "new organ" is a paradigm shift for medicine. Hopefully it will usher in renewed interest in human nutrition and its impact on our health.

Using the knowledge I gained from William Davis and David Perlmutter I realized that we have the opportunity to eliminate many human diseases. This article focuses on diabetes:

Eliminating Diabetes – Diseases of Malnutrition

Desert Health
October 2015

Diabetes mellitus is a group of diseases that have in common an elevated blood sugar. They are disorders of carbohydrate metabolism. Emerging scientific evidence points to malnutrition, not the starvation type, but rather eating the wrong foods, as the dominant cause of diabetes. There is a genetic component to developing diabetes, but this is small in comparison to the impact of nutrition. The frequency of diabetes has increased exponentially since 1980 along with the increase in overweight and obesity due to what we eat.

This article describes the impact of what we eat on the development of both type 1 and type 2 diabetes. Diabetes that develops during pregnancy, gestational diabetes, will be lumped with type 2 diabetes because they have essentially the same mechanisms that result in high blood sugar. The information in this article draws mainly from the work of two physicians, William Davis (*Wheat Belly* and *Wheat Belly Total Health*) and David Perlmutter (*Grain Brain* and *Brain Maker*).

As a group, the diseases of diabetes have a tremendous impact on the health of Americans causing heart disease, stroke, organ failure, blindness, neuropathy, dementia and premature death. Collectively we spend more money treating diabetes than any other group of diseases including cancer and heart disease. Eliminating diabetes, or making it very rare, would be an enormous benefit to our collective health. This may seem far-fetched but eliminating diabetes is easily within our reach. All we need to do is to eat the right foods.

Inside the body, the mechanisms of diabetes are highly complex. Drugs used to treat diabetes attempt to manipulate these mechanisms. However, the triggers of diabetes are not complex. Unfortunately, they remain largely hidden in plain sight.

Inflammatory proteins – Auto-immunity – Type 1 Diabetes

Type 1 diabetes is one of many auto-immune diseases that rob us of our health. In the case of type 1 diabetes, we form antibodies that attack and destroy the cells in the pancreas that make insulin. Without insulin we cannot metabolize sugar and we die. All type 1 diabetics must take insulin to live. The complications of type 1 diabetes even treated with insulin include reduced circulation to many parts of the body, blindness, kidney failure, neuropathy and heart disease. Without optimal treatment, people with type 1 diabetes die prematurely.

What causes us to form these auto-antibodies that destroy our own tissues? For years this was thought to be due to viruses that reprogram our DNA. We now know that "leaky gut" from food substances, mainly proteins, get into blood stream and are considered foreign by our immune system. We form antibodies against these proteins, a type of inflammatory reaction, that also attack and destroy our tissues, in this case the insulin-making cells of our pancreas.

Where do these inflammatory proteins come from? Mainly from eating grains such as wheat and other foods made with flour. Grains such wheat and oats contain prolamin proteins, such as the gluten protein complex, that are inflammatory to the human body and increase intestinal permeability or "leaky gut". It appears to be that the entire spectrum of auto-immune disease, hypothyroidism, rheumatoid arthritis and other inflammatory arthritis, multiple sclerosis and other neurodegenerative diseases, and many allergies are the result of eating inflammatory proteins. These diseases are for the most part unique to humans and are not seen in the animal kingdom.

Excess carbohydrates – Increased body fat – Type 2 and Gestational Diabetes

Body fat is much more than the storage of energy. Fat is hormonally active in the body and causes inflammation and changes in carbohydrate metabolism. While genetics play a role in susceptibility, there is a level of body fat that would result in almost everyone developing type 2 diabetes.

What causes increased body fat? We now understand it is not from the fatty foods we eat. In general fats satisfy us and reduce hunger. Increased body fat comes mainly from eating carbohydrates -- grains, sweets and alcohol that drive up hunger and cause us to eat more. Carbohydrates and fat are energy foods and the body will try to use the carbohydrates first. All the excess carbohydrates we consume that are not used for energy are stored as body fat through a mechanism called lipogenesis.

Carbohydrates are sugars and starches and come mainly from grains and sweets. Starches such as grains are simply chains of sugar. The amount of sugar in a carbohydrate food is called the glycemic load. It turns out the grains such as the wheat in bread, muffins, cookies, cakes and pizza crust have the highest glycemic load along with sweets such as ice cream.

During pregnancy women eat much more and if excess carbohydrates are consumed, gestational diabetes is often the result, putting the baby and the mother at risk.

You are what you eat

This old phrase has new meanings now that the gut microbiome, the 100 trillion organisms in our intestines that determine much of our health, is being understood. Eating the whole foods of nature -- nuts, vegetables, fruit, seeds, healthy fish and meat, results in a healthy gut flora and healthy intestines. Diabetes would be very rare if this is all we ate. Inflammatory proteins and excess sugars result in an unhealthy gut flora, leaky gut, inflammation and a staggering burden of disease, including the diseases of diabetes. Stop this malnutrition and we can stop diabetes.

My journey into healthy nutrition and greater wellness is far from over. Life is a journey and I plan to stay active and contribute to the knowledge of wellness as long as I can, which hopefully will be a long time. We have just begun to understand the real impact nutrition has on our health.

Terry Wahls, MD is a physician everyone should know about and study. Her protocol, painstakingly developed and written to reverse her own and others multiple sclerosis, is a blueprint for healthy nutrition. I consider her book the "state of the art" for controlling or reversing auto-immune disease and maintaining high level wellness. I wrote the following book review coming out in *Family Medicine*.

The Wahls Protocol

Terry Wahls, MD.
Penguin Group. 2014.

This is an important book. Terry Wahls is a Clinical Professor of Medicine at the University of Iowa. In her 40s she developed disabling multiple sclerosis (MS). Despite the latest medical treatments her disease progressed. She undertook painstaking research into what nutritional and other lifestyle factors might help her with the disease. By adopting an anti-inflammatory Paleo styled diet she was able to reverse her autoimmune disease and return to normal function. Since then she has reached out to help others suffering from MS and other autoimmune conditions in a variety of clinical trials. She conducts a clinic at the University of Iowa, has an interactive website,[1] and lectures widely. She has met with considerable success helping others and this book is a culmination of her work to date.

Wahls is a serious medical scientist. She has 25 peer reviewed publications on PubMed. She approaches her work in autoimmune disease biologically and provides strong arguments for both nutritional causes of these diseases and nutritional healing.

The Wahls Protocol is a manual for patients and a great introduction to nutritional and lifestyle healing for clinicians. The book is divided into three parts: Before You Get Started, Eating for Cellular Health, and Going Beyond Food. Nutrition is the centerpiece of *The Wahls Protocol*. She gives patients three options, each building on the other in levels of intensity.

The Wahls Diet (level one) is a type of Paleo diet and she goes into detail in describing its specificity. There is no gluten, no dairy, no eggs and few if any legumes. There are 9 cups of vegetables and whole fruits daily and she is very specific on these:

- Three cups raw or cooked leafy greens such as kale, collards, chards, Asian greens and dark lettuces

- Three cups deeply colored vegetables and fruits, such as berries, tomatoes, beets, carrots and squash

- Three cups sulfur-rich vegetables, such as broccoli, cabbage, asparagus, Brussels sprouts, turnips, radishes, onions, and garlic

While she is supportive of being vegetarian for personal choice, she does not recommend it. She goes into detail why she thinks food from animal sources is important, and her diet includes grass-fed meat and wild caught meat and fish.

The Wahls Paleo diet (level two) is the same as above with these added components:

- Reduce or eliminate all non-gluten grains, legumes and potatoes

- Add seaweed or algae, and organ meats

- Add fermented foods such as sauerkraut, pickles, kimchi and kombucha tea

She describes why these additions will add to the anti-inflammatory nature of the diet.

The Wahls Paleo Plus diet (level three) makes these additions and modifications to the above:

- Eliminate all grains, legumes and potatoes

- Reduce the cups of vegetables and whole fruit to 6 cups daily

- Add coconut oil and full-fat coconut milk

- Eat just twice daily and fast twelve to sixteen hours every day and night

Other lifestyle factors presented by Dr. Wahls are reducing the toxic load in the environment, exercise, stress management and the mental health aspects of recovery. She emphasizes getting nutrients from food and not supplements. She does recommend vitamin D, calcium, magnesium, Omega-3 fatty acids, coenzyme Q and dietary enzymes.

Obviously this is all based on empiric evidence and is a work in progress. It is becoming clear that an anti-inflammatory diet is real, and people do respond biologically to these principles.

This book should be read by all primary care clinicians and by medical students and residents. Any patient with multiple sclerosis deserves to be aware of and consider taking this option, even connecting with Dr. Wahls. Patients with other autoimmune diseases may benefit also.

Biologic understandings of how nutrition both causes disease and its power to heal are rapidly emerging. This is part of the new biology and deserves to be much more widely researched and taught.

Dysbiosis is the new diagnostic term that underlies many gastrointestinal problems, such as acid reflux and irritable bowel disease. Dysbiosis is the name for an unhealthy gut microbiome that is causing health problems in the host person. Extreme dysbiosis is most likely the basis for serious inflammatory bowel diseases, such as ulcerative colitis and Crohn's disease. This research article review validates the work of Dr. Terry Wahls.

Does Dysbiosis Cause Multiple Sclerosis?

Internal Medicine Alert
June 30, 2016;38(12):91-92

Synopsis: Increasing evidence suggests that dysbiosis, a disorder in the gut microbiome, leads to autoimmune diseases, including multiple sclerosis.

Source: Glenn JD, Mowry EM. Emerging concepts on the gut microbiome and multiple sclerosis. J Interferon Cytokine Research. 2016;36:347-357.

Two scientists from the Department of Neurology at Johns Hopkins University School of Medicine recently reviewed the emerging science of the human gut microbiome and the development of autoimmune diseases, particularly multiple sclerosis. The gut microbiome has complex bidirectional interactions with the human immune system.

While the bacteria in the human gut has the highest density ever recorded in any ecosystem, there are even more viruses in the gut, most importantly the bacteriophages that infect the bacteria and exchange DNA.

The microbiome develops at birth and is enhanced by both vaginal delivery and breastfeeding. Children born by Cesarean section have a delay in their microbiome development as do children not breastfed. These changes have been reported for up to 7 years. Multiple sclerosis patients feature a higher rate of C-section birth and shorter duration of breastfeeding than controls.[1-2]

There is emerging evidence leading researchers to believe that dysbiosis, disorders in the gut microbiome, form a biological basis for the development of autoimmune diseases. Some of the strongest evidence exists for Crohn's disease and multiple sclerosis.[3,4] The Western diet, with its unhealthy trans fats, excessive sugar, and inflammatory proteins, has been associated with dysbiosis.

Commentary

The number of books being written by physicians and biologists on the gut microbiome has exploded in the last few years.[5-8] Compelling evidence says our health depends on what we eat in profound ways, with the gut microbiome acting as a critical intermediary. Disorder in the gut microbiome has become the leading theory behind the development of autoimmune diseases.

Terry Wahls is an internist at the University of Iowa who developed disabling multiple sclerosis in 2002. Conventional therapy, including new biologic agents, were ineffective in halting the progression of her disease. After years of research into scientific articles, she adopted an anti-inflammatory diet that over time halted and then reversed her disease and she is now fully functional. She has an ongoing clinical trial at the University of Iowa and she has helped hundreds of other multiple sclerosis patients. Her 2014 book, *The Wahls Protocol*, describes her therapeutic approach in detail.[9]

The human microbiome exists throughout the body with 70% of the organisms residing in our gut. Research into its many functions in health and disease are early in their development. It is likely that an understanding of the interactions and effects of the microbiome on our bodies will profoundly change medical practice in the years to come.

Dr. Mark Hyman, the most recognized leader in Functional Medicine, has a new book on why eating a diet of mostly healthy fats from natural foods is best. This well-referenced book takes our nutrition full circle and buries the low fat food paradigm. My book review will be published in *Family Medicine* after this book goes to print.

Eat Fat, Get Thin

Mark Hyman, MD
New York: Little, Brown and Company, 2016

Mark Hyman trained in family medicine and is a major figure in the emerging area called Functional Medicine. He is chair and director of the Cleveland Clinic Center for Functional Medicine, and is chairman of the Institute for Functional Medicine. Of his previous sixteen books, the most noteworthy is *The Blood Sugar Solution* (2012).[1] With *Eat Fat, Get Thin* Hyman presents a more positive message about what to eat (healthy fats) rather than emphasizing what not to eat (high glycemic carbohydrates).

Hyman joins a growing list of physician authors putting to rest the mistaken recommendation made over four decades to eat a low fat diet.[2-4] Not all fats are healthy and some are toxic, such as the trans fats in processed foods. The content of the book can be predicted by the cover containing an avocado, tree nuts, olive oil and some dark chocolate.

Hyman details how excess body fat comes mainly from the ingestion of high amounts of carbohydrates.[1-4] Carbohydrates cause the release of insulin that result in blood sugar fluctuations that drive hunger. Excess carbohydrates are converted to fat in the liver through lipogenesis.

Some interesting facts are presented here. The Joslin Diabetes Center at Harvard was named after Dr. Elliott P. Joslin, who in the 1920s recommended a diet of 75% fat, 20% protein and 5% carbohydrates to treat diabetes. After fat become demonized starting in the 1950s, the carbohydrate recommendation went up to 60%. Hyman reports that currently researchers at the Joslin Diabetes Center are once again recommending a diet high in fat, up to 70%, for the treatment of type 2 diabetes.[5]

The strength of this book is an extensive analysis of what constitutes healthy fats, mostly from plant sources. Hyman gives a detailed explanation as to why he thinks that some fats from animal sources, eggs, grass fed beef or free range poultry, and wild caught fish, are important for healthy nutrition. He promotes what he calls the "Pegan

Diet", mostly Vegan but some amount of healthy Paleo foods.

I find that patients like this book recommendation because of its positive title and message. Students and residents will find it an informative and entertaining read, and will be helped in changing away from the paradigm of low fat foods. All of the information is sound and well referenced. For a more in depth scientific analysis of why we should avoid high glycemic carbohydrates, I recommend Harvard's David Ludwig and his recently published book, *Always Hungry?* (2016).[6]

The following article reinforces the science that eating saturated fat from healthy sources is good for you.

Welcome Back, Saturated Fat

Internal Medicine Alert
June 15, 2016

Synopsis: The NIH has been conducting systematic reviews and meta-analyses of randomized controlled trials that show replacing saturated fat with unsaturated vegetable oils rich in linoleic acid does not result in a reduction in atherosclerosis, cardiovascular morbidity, and death.

Source: Ransden CE, Daisy EZ, Majchirak-Hong S, et al. Re-evaluation of the traditional diet-heart hypothesis: Analysis of recovered data from the Minnesota Coronary

Experiment (1968-73). BMJ 2016;353:i1246.

A team of investigators from the National Institutes of Health has been conducting systemic reviews and meta-analyses of previously published and unpublished data from experiments testing the traditional diet-heart hypothesis that saturated fat contributes to cardiovascular disease and death. This hypothesis and subsequent dietary recommendations were based on evidence that replacing saturated fat with unsaturated vegetable oils, particularly with linoleic acid, lowered serum cholesterol.[1,2] At the same time, observational studies showed that lower serum cholesterol was associated with lower cardiovascular morbidly and mortality.[3] The authors report that no randomized controlled trials of using unsaturated fats to lower cardiovascular morbidity have been conducted to prove the hypothesis.

The Minnesota Coronary Experiment was conducted between 1968 and 1973 in one nursing home and six state mental hospitals. Researches randomized 9,423 women and men ranging in age from 20 to 97, with a mean age of 52. One-quarter of the subjects were ≥65 of age. Feeding subjects in a cafeteria allowed for more precise assurance of diet adherence than most population diet studies. Both groups ate a similar amount of fat and the average body mass index was 24.5 kg/m. In the intervention group, saturated fat in cooking oils, salad dressings, and butter was replaced with corn oil products and corn oil polyunsaturated margarine. Autopsy data was available on 149 subjects.

The intervention group with more unsaturated fat intake had significant reductions in both total and low-density lipoprotein (LDL) cholesterol, an average of 13.8%. However, there no difference in mortality among any age or sex cohort. The intervention group actually had a higher number of cardiovascular infarcts. Autopsy reports showed no difference in degree of atherosclerosis among the two groups.

The same authors previously reported a re-analysis of unpublished data from another large randomized controlled trial, the Sidney Diet Heart Study conducted during the same period. In this study the intervention group on the unsaturated fat diet (linoleic acid from vegetable oils) actually showed a higher cardiovascular morbidity and mortality.[4]

Commentary

It is becoming clear that saturated fats from natural food sources are not a cause of cardiovascular disease. Indeed, the opposite may be true as discussed by Dr. Mark Hyman in his new book, *Eat Fat, Get Thin*.[5] The authors in this study noted that any food consumed is a substance that is biochemically processed in the human body. Man has consumed saturated fats for thousands of years and most commercially available unsaturated fats are processed foods foreign to the body. The fact that LDL particles in the unsaturated fat group have greater LDL particle oxidation and are more inflammatory to the cardiovascular system may explain the paradox that lowering total and LDL cholesterol did not result in health benefits.

A recent randomized, controlled trial showed patients on a low carbohydrate/high-fat diet had increased LDL particle size (less inflammatory) than patients eating a traditional American Heart Association low-fat diet with higher complex carbohydrates, whose LDL particles actually shrank and become more inflammatory.[6] Hence measuring only total and LDL cholesterol has limitations in that such measurements do not show how inflammatory these cholesterol particles are.

It has become apparent that clinicians have been giving wrong dietary advice to patients for many decades. The low-fat and non-fat food industry was a mistake because it resulted in higher carbohydrate intake and coincided with the epidemic of overweight, obesity and type 2 diabetes, major risk factors for cardiovascular disease.

Science has a way of breaking paradigms and keeping us humble. Greater understanding of the biochemistry of nutrition and the human body gives healthcare providers an opportunity to have better nutrition recommendations and hopefully, improved food science. The relative lack of nutrition education in American medicine is most unfortunate, as nutrition is emerging as a major therapeutic tool to prevent and reverse disease.

CONCLUSIONS

I hope this book has convinced you that following a low carbohydrate diet focusing on the foods of nature is the healthiest way to eat. Carbohydrate is the macronutrient that our body actually does not need since we can manufacture glucose from fat and protein. Some carbohydrate from whole fruit, vegetables, nuts and seeds is fine and contributes to an optimal diet. Healthy fats, such as in nuts, seeds, vegetables, olive and coconut oil, wild caught meat and fish supply us with all the energy we need to thrive. Proteins, the building blocks of life, should also be obtained from these sources. Cultivating grains is a mistake the human race made starting ten thousand years ago, and the burden of disease caused by the inflammatory proteins in grains is staggering. Processed foods with hybridization and genetic modification have resulted in grains being more toxic, added sugars and the harmful effects of high fructose corn syrup. Food science needs to hit the reset button!

There are many inconvenient truths facing the human race today. Al Gore gave us greater awareness of the impact of climate change, accelerated by our lack of caring for our planet. Many of our societies have fallen victim to entropy, greater disorganization and violence. The inconvenient truth in nutrition is that we have created a remarkably unhealthy diet. What we thought was healthy for decades turns out to be wrong.

The anthropologist and physiologist Jared Diamond declared in 1999 in *Discover* magazine that becoming farmers was the worst mistake in the history of the human race. Evidence shows that we were much healthier as hunter/gatherers with greater height, stronger bones, and better teeth just to mention a few findings. This truth is the basis for the Paleolitihic Diet (Paleo for short) originally described by gastroenterologist Walter Voegtlin in the 1970s. Loren Cordain made the diet popular with is 2002 book, *The Paleo Diet*.

I would never say that all farming is bad. Farming is essential for sustaining our population. Many healthy foods come from farms, and shopping healthy today often means visits to a local farmer's market. Eating locally grown foods, or the farm to table concept, is one of the best ways to eat healthy.

So far food science at major American universities, heavily funded by the food industry, may have caused us harm as they try to do well. We have genetically modified many foods without regard for the impact on our complex physiology, including the gut microbiome. William Davis in *Wheat Belly* goes into detail about modern 42 chromosome wheat engineered by hybridization at the University of Minnesota by Norman Borlag who died a great hero. We are paying the price of the unintended consequences of this wheat compared with the 14 chromosome einkorn natural wheat. Even though wheat is inflammatory, if you insist on having foods made from flour use one from nuts or seeds as shown in the recipes in Appendix V. Food science must become much more sophisticated as it attempts to genetically modify the foods of nature. We do that at our potential benefit and peril.

I continue to speak and write on nutrition and a healthy lifestyle. In my mid-60s my lifestyle and medical practice has changed more than any time previous. I plan to stay lean and fit and hope to inspire my patients and readers of this book to do also. Please join the Lean and Fit community on our website, www.leanandfitlife.com. I offer professional coaching and advice for your journey to become lean and fit. We have so much more to learn and have within our power to develop the healthiest humans that have ever lived.

APPENDICES

Appendix I

Suggested Daily Meal Plan

Healthy nutrition does not require counting calories, even if you want to lose weight. By eating a diet high in fat and protein from healthy sources, the appetite is greatly reduced resulting in eating fewer calories naturally. Limited carbohydrates, and eating only those in natural foods, does not result in the unstable blood sugar common among those eating grains, sweets and drinking excessive alcohol. Here is a typical daily meal plan I follow:

Breakfast

My bowl no longer contains cereal, rather:

1. A handful of tree nuts (almonds, walnuts, pecans, cashew nuts or Brazil nuts) Mix and match as you like for variety.
2. A layer of berries, usually fresh blueberries but sometimes strawberries, raspberries or blackberries, or as back-up dried cranberries. About ¼ cup.
3. Four heaping tablespoons of plain yogurt with live cultures, preferably goat milk or coconut milk. Will settle for cow's milk if that is all that is available. Alternative or in addition some Kefir, another fermented food.
4. A layer of ground flaxseed, chia seeds or hemp seeds.

5. Unsweetened almond milk or coconut milk for added moisture. Will use whole cow's milk if that is all that is available.

Two eggs, hard boiled or fried in butter.

After these high protein foods, I may have a banana and/or an orange. The sugar in these fruits is absorbed more slowly after eating protein.

Water, coffee or tea are the best beverages during the day.

This hearty breakfast will nourish me even with hard work for 5-6 hours.

Lunch

A salad, preferably a spinach salad with other vegetables (especially avocado and tomatoes), nuts, berries and a protein such as shrimp, salmon or chicken breast. No croutons!

Water, coffee or tea.

Dinner

An entrée source of protein such as wild salmon, scallops or other fish. If meat, eat a modest portion of grass fed beef such as a petit filet, lamb, pork, chicken or turkey. I eat fish two times to one over meat.

Healthy vegetables such as garlic spinach, asparagus, broccoli, squash or yams, carrots, tomatoes. Sometimes natural whole or Rosemary potatoes. Whole potatoes are a starch but they have many nutrients and my exercise is able to compensate for carbohydrate load. Sometimes I eat vegetarian and my entre is eggplant.

Water and one glass of red wine (other alcohol may be used but avoid the grains such as wheat in beer). An ultra-light beer is acceptable, as is white wine.

A modest amount of dark chocolate may be taken for dessert with the glass of wine. Look for at least 70% cocoa.

This meal plan does not require any snacking, and snacking is to be avoided. If an afternoon snack is desired, I recommend an apple.

Put 8-12 hour fasting periods into your day and night eating schedule. Fasting is very healthy for your metabolism and is much easier when fat and protein are the mainstay of your diet.

Appendix II

Supplements

This will be a short section because supplements play very little role in promoting and maintaining human health. There are a few exceptions as stated below.

I often tell patients that "good health does not come in a bottle". That glib comment is backed up by science. With rare exception, controlled research trials looking at the use of vitamins and other supplements compared with just good food show that the supplements do not add health benefit, and may cause harm.

I like the expression of Colin Campbell in his book, *Whole,* that supplements confuse the body. We evolved to the foods of nature, not to take a bolus of one or a batch of supplements in doses that are not represented in food.

Gerard Mullin in his book, *The Gut Balance Revolution,* uses the metaphor of food as a symphony. He points out that using supplements is like taking a few musicians out of the symphony and asking them to play comparable music. It does not happen.

There is one exception worth noting. Evolution did not care if we lived past our child bearing years. Vitamin D is a hormone like substance we manufacture in our skin from sunlight. Vitamin D is vital to many body functions, not just our bones. It is not present in natural foods but is sometimes added to dairy products. When we age, our skin's ability to make vitamin D from sunlight wanes and many people over age 50 become deficient in Vitamin D even if they are in the sun. This is especially true of seniors over age 65. Hence, Vitamin D is the one vitamin that should be taken by mature adults. Vitamin D3 is the digestible form and 2000 – 5000 IU should be taken daily. This will provide an optimal level of Vitamin D in the blood between 40 and 60 (the normal range of Vitamin D listed in most labs is between 30 and 100).

The only other supplement I take is a mixture of glucosamine, chondroitin and MSM. This does not treat arthritis, but may have some role in preventing the loss of cartilage that leads to arthritis in our joints, especially the knees. The necessary dosage is unknown but I take one of the readily available products that have these three ingredients as recommended on the bottle.

Vegans and some seniors especially over the age of 80 become deficient in Vitamin B12. This can easily be tested for in a blood test. If the need is there, take 1 mg or 1000 mcg of Vitamin B12 daily. B12 shots are not necessary even for someone who has pernicious anemia. Enough of the daily oral vitamin will suffice.

Lots of people ask me about fish oil and omega-3 fatty acids. These are very important and are best obtained by eating fish a few times a week, especially salmon. Taken as a supplement they have not been shown to offer a health benefit and may even raise the rate of certain cancers.

Some supplements are food products such as saw palmetto and grape seed extract. These are very expensive ways to get a small amount of what is readily available in healthy foods.

Forget that once a day multi-vitamin. It will not prevent you from catching colds or getting sick. Eat real health foods, especially the "Superfoods" as listed next.

Some of the authors I recommend cite a limited number of supplements, such as David Perlmutter in *Grain Brain* and *Brain Maker*. I do not object to these but I do not take them so they are not listed here. I shun authors who promote lots of supplements and most of them have a conflict of interest since they sell them on their websites. I strive to get my patients off an excessive list of expensive supplements. Better to use your money to buy healthy food!

Appendix III

Superfoods

I have listed here foods that have been shown to be the healthiest foods we can eat. They are listed alphabetically and if you include many of these in your daily nutrition you will be enhancing your health every day.

There are many "superfood" lists and they include what is here and sometimes more, such as the book by Jonny Bowden in Appendix IV. I like this shorter list of the best of the good foods. If a food of nature is not listed here, do not feel that it must be avoided. Remember, eat the foods of nature and you will be better off than the great majority of the population.

1. Almonds, raw
2. Almond Milk, unsweetened
3. Apples
4. Asparagus
5. Avocados
6. Bananas
7. Beans, black, pinto & garbanzo
8. Bell Peppers, yellow, green, red & orange
9. Beets
10. Blackberries
11. Blueberries
12. Broccoli
13. Brussels Sprouts
14. Carrots
15. Cheese
16. Cherries

17. Chicken
18. Coconut Milk, unsweetened
19. Coconut Oil
20. Cranberries
21. Eggs
22. Herring
23. Honeydew
24. Kale
25. Kiwi
26. Lemons
27. Lentils
28. Limes
29. Olives
30. Olive Oil
31. Oranges
32. Peaches
33. Peas
34. Plums
35. Pomegranates
36. Raspberries
37. Red Grapes
38. Spinach
39. Strawberries
40. Tea
41. Tofu
42. Tomatoes
43. Turmeric
44. Tuna
45. Turkey
46. Walnuts
47. Water
48. Wild Salmon
49. Yams & Sweet Potatoes
50. Yogurt, unsweetened

Appendix IV

Recommended Reading

William Davis, *Wheat Belly* (2011) and *Wheat Belly Total Health* (2014). Both by Rodale.

Dr. Davis is a cardiologist who got me started after I read *Wheat Belly* in 2013 and became free of grains. His books are well referenced and he is the champion of a grain free lifestyle. Dr. Davis reversed his own type 2 diabetes and developed extraordinarily healthy lipids from following this approach to eating. He is a modern day Robert Atkins, another cardiologist who healed himself before healing others.

David Perlmutter, *Grain Brain* (2013) and *Brain Maker* (2015). Both by Little, Brown & Co.

Dr. Perlmutter is a neurologist with an advanced degree in nutrition. *Grain Brain* built off of William Davis's *Wheat Belly* and emphasized how high blood sugar and the inflammatory effects of grains cause a host of neurodegenerative diseases including Alzheimer's disease. *Brain Maker* is a breakthrough book bringing the emerging science about the crucial role of the gut microbiome in health and disease, a new "organ" that totally depends on what we eat. An unhealthy gut microbiome, induced by grains, causes leaky gut and most auto-immune diseases and neurodegeneration.

Daniel Lieberman, *The Story of the Human Body: Evolution, Health and Disease* (2013). Vintage Books.

This Harvard evolutionary biologist knows more about health, nutrition and disease than most physicians. He describes in detail how the nutrition of our paleolitihic ancestors was much healthier than our processed foods today. Most modern processed food is "mismatch" with our evolutionary body and he described how we are in a state of "disevolution". This is a powerful call for revolutionary change by a brilliant academic.

Terry Wahls. *The Wahls Protocol* (2014). Avery (Penguin Group.

Terry Wahls is a professor of internal medicine at the University of Iowa. At the peak of her career she developed disabling multiple sclerosis (MS). After failing to improve on both standard and new experimental medications, she sought relief through healthy nutrition and lifestyle. An anti-inflammatory low carbohydrate Paleo diet reversed her disease and she is back at work and lecturing widely (See her TED talk and YouTube presentations). She has an ongoing clinical trial helping others to reverse MS and other auto-immune disease. Anyone suffering from such problems, or even persons wanting to avoid such diseases, should read this book and follow the protocol. She has three levels of diet depending on how intense a person wants to be with their nutrition.

Jeff Volek & Stephen Phinney. *The Art and Science of Low Carbohydrate Living* (2011) and *The Art and Science of Low Carbohydrate Performance* (2012). Both by Beyond Obesity, LLC.

Jeff Volek, RD, PhD is an academic nutritionist at The Ohio State University and Stephen Phinney, MD, PhD recently retired from the food science department at the University of California, Davis. They provide the hard science behind the benefits of low carbohydrate nutrition. In their book on performance, they describe how great endurance athletes such as the tennis player, Novak Djokovic, excel without eating carbohydrates except for what is in whole foods. Being a fat burner during long athletic events results in a steady blood sugar and steady performance compared with athletes that get tired, dizzy or cramp when they bottom out their limited supply of carbohydrates.

T. Colin Campbell & Howard Jacobson. *Whole: Rethinking the Science of Nutrition* (2013). BenBella Books.

Colin Campbell is a distinguished nutrition scientist at Cornell (now emeritus). His research focused on nutrition and cancer and he conducted the largest epidemiologic research in the world showing that cancer and animal protein are strongly associated. He is a champion of a whole food plant based diet (vegan). He first published *The China Study* in 2006 and *Whole* summarizes those findings and provides a critique of how most nutrition science falls short in providing the information we need due to attempting to study single nutrients rather than whole foods. He also describes how the food industry in America is suppressing vital information about healthy and unhealthy foods.

Rick Warren, Daniel Amen & Mark Hyman. *The Daniel Plan: 40 Days to a Healthier Life* (2013). Zondervan.

Rick Warren was an overweight pastor in Orange County, CA and decided he had better lose weight and become healthy. Rather than do that himself he challenged his congregation to join him. He enlisted the help of two physicians, Daniel Amen, a psychiatrist who has shown through imaging studies that the higher the blood sugar the more rapid the brain atrophy, and Mark Hyman, a family physician who advised Bill Clinton on becoming healthier by giving up grains and processed food. This book covers how in 40 days the congregation of Warren's church lost over a hundred thousand pounds. Rick Warren provides spiritual advice while the doctors advise on healthy nutrition.

Denise Minger. *Death by Food Pyramid: How Shoddy Science, Sketchy Politics and Shady Special Interests Have Ruined Our Health... and How to Reclaim It* (2013). Primal Blueprint Publishing.

Denise Minger is a super-smart self-taught data junkie and in this book lays bare food politics in America and what is healthy nutrition. She dissects each of the recommended diets in America from the four food groups through the pyramids. She also reanalyzed the data from Colin Campbell's *The China Study* showing that, among other things, fish from wild sources was also associated with lower cancer rates.

Scott Jurek. *Eat & Run: My Unlikely Journey to Ultramarathon Greatness* (2012). Houghton Mifflin Harcourt Publishing.

Scott Jurek is the first male star performer of ultramarathons. He is also a vegan. This book is his life story from his childhood near Duluth Minnesota to setting new records in the Western States 100-mile Endurance Run winning it six years in a row. His journey of being lean and fit is inspiring and he continues to break limits just setting a new record for completing the Appalachian Trail in 46 days.

Dan Buetner. *The Blue Zones Solution: Eating and Living Like the World's Healthiest People* (2015). National Geographic Society.

Who can argue about the food ingredients of the healthiest people on Earth? What I find fascinating about the nutrition of the Blue Zone populations is that they are mostly very healthy and the people are lean and fit and relaxed. Most do eat some of the toxic carbohydrates such as breads. They live an average of eight years longer than other populations. I wonder how long they would live with optimal nutrition without the inflammatory foods?

Justin Sonnenburg, PhD and Erica Sonnenburg. PhD. *The Good Gut: Taking Control of Your Weight, Your Mood, and Your Long Term Health (2015)* Penguin Press.

This husband and wife team are both microbiologists at Stanford University and are leading researchers in the human gut microbiome. They wrote this book for the general public in order to spread the word about the importance of the gut microbiome in human health. Their lack of medical training gives the book some limitations, however they provide lots of important information and validate the academic credibility of work in improving the gut microbiome, a critical "organ" for human health.

Gerard Mullin, MD. *The Gut Balance Revolution: Boost Your Metablism, Restore Your Inner Ecology, and Lose the Weight for Good!* (2015). Rodale, Inc.

Dr. Mullin is a gastroenterologist at Johns Hopkins University School of Medicine. He tells his childhood story of being embarrassingly fat once weighing over 300 pounds. He studied nutrition to lose the weight and as a medical scientist learned the critical importance of how human nutrition feeds the gut microbiome to not only help us lose weight, but also to be healthy overall. His largely self-developed diet plan is mostly consistent with what is presented in this book. However, he is not fully grain free in his recommendations, a limitation that can be overlooked by the strength of his overall recommendations. Being from one of the world's most prestigious medical schools, he provides academic credibility to what is presented here.

Robynne Chutkin, MD. *Gutbliss* (2013) and *The Microbiome Solution* (2015). Both by Penguin Group.

Dr. Chutkin is a gastroenterologist specializing in women's health. She uses nutrition to correct both common and uncommon GI problems such as bloating, acid reflux, irritable bowel syndrome, and inflammatory bowel disease (Crohn's disease and ulcerative colitis). While her recommendations apply to men and women, her writing style and testimonials will resonate very well with women.

David Ludwig, MD, PhD. *Always Hungry?* (2016). Grand Central Life & Style (Hachette Book Group).

Dr. Ludwig is a pediatric endocrinologist at Harvard with impeccable academic credentials. His new book for the public reinforces the problems of excess carbohydrates and processed foods. He gives the low carbohydrate approach to nutrition solid academic credibility and also provides practical solutions. Many will like his maintenance diet but I consider it too high in carbohydrates (50%). He also only addresses weight and does not consider the role of inflammatory proteins such as in grains.

Robert Lustig, MD. *Fat Chance* (2012). Penguin Group.

Dr. Lustig is a pediatric endocrinologist at the University of California, San Francisco. He is best known for his attack on sugar and high fructose corn syrup added to most processed foods. He makes a strong case that these sugars are causing the global epidemic of overweight and obesity and that only radical public health measures will save us from spiraling into obesity and poor health. While his focus is limited to sugars, his message is powerful and the science is excellent.

Mark Hyman. *Eat Fat, Get Thin* (2016). Little, Brown and Company.

Mark Hyman is a family physician and the director of the Cleveland Clinic Center for Functional Medicine. He is also the chairman of the Institute for Functional Medicine. With *Eat Fat, Get Thin* Hyman puts a positive spin on healthy nutrition by discussing what we can eat rather than what we must give up. A clue to the book is on the cover, with an avocado, tree nuts, olive oil and dark chocolate, not bacon.

JJ Virgin. *The Virgin Diet* (2012), HarperCollins and *JJ Virgin's Sugar Impact Diet* (2014) Hachette Book Group.

JJ Virgin is a nutrition and fitness coach who became a bestselling author. Her first book eliminates the unhealthy processed and carbohydrate foods. Her second book is useful in that it identifies the hidden sugars in many foods that can prevent weight loss in someone thinking they are eating right. Along with Robynne Chutkin and Terry Wahls, this book would be especially useful to women.

Jonny Bowden. *The 150 Healthiest Foods on Earth.* (2007) Fair Winds Press, Beverly, MA.

For anyone who thinks my list of 50 foods is too limiting, this book is a very comprehensive description of 150 superfoods of nature. Many of the high glycemic fruits are listed but as long as one remembers the use of whole fruits in moderation because of the sugars, this book will be very useful.

Websites:

www.leanandfitlife.com by Joseph Scherger, MD
www.cureality.com by William Davis, MD
www.drperlmutter.com by David Perlmutter, MD
www.drhyman.com by Mark Hyman, MD
www.rawfoodsos.com by Denise Minger

Appendix V

Recipes

My friend and patient Barbara Rogers read *Lean and Fit* and quickly lost what little extra weight she had. She felt so much better. As someone who loves to cook, she started writing recipes based on the nutrition presented here. On her own and at her own expense, she brought to my office bounded copies of her many recipes under the title, Healthier Way of Life. A range of these recipes is presented here. Many more recipes from Barbara Rogers may be found on our website, www.leanandfitlife.com and on her website, www.itsanograinerlife.com.

Thank you Barbara!

Healthier Way of Life by Barbara Rogers

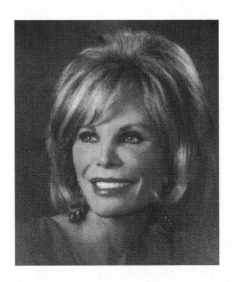

Hot Cereal Using Almond Butter, Nuts and Seeds

Ingredients:

⅓ cup unsweetened almond or coconut milk
2 tbsp. flaxseeds, raw
3 tbsp. pecans, raw, chopped, may use another nut
3 tbsp. walnuts, raw, chopped, may use another nut
2 tbsp. sunflower seeds, raw
2 to 3 tbsp. almond butter

Directions:

Mix all in a bowl/cup and heat in a microware all ingredients about 50 seconds or until warm.

Green Chili Egg Casserole

Preheat oven to 400 degrees, 200 C

Ingredients:

½ cup butter, melted
1 (16 oz.) cottage cheese
1 lb. shredded Monterey Jack cheese
2 (4 oz.) cans diced green chilies
1 tsp. baking powder
10 eggs
¼ cup coconut flour
½ tsp. salt
¾ cup either grass fed ground beef, turkey or Italian
    sausage (optional)

Directions:

Grease a 6x10-inch pan with the ½ cup melted butter. Mix cottage cheese, Jack cheese, green chilies, eggs, baking powder, salt, meat (if using) and coconut flour together in a bowl. Then pour mixture into the greased 6x10-inch pan. Bake in the preheated oven for 15 minutes at 400 degrees. Then reduce heat to 350 degrees F (175 degrees C); bake until middle of casserole is set, about 50 more minutes. Allow to stand for 10 minutes before serving.

Note: This dish freezes exceptionally well. Unprocessed ground Italian sausage (without the casing), ham and turkey can be found at Sprouts and Whole Foods markets. Sauté the meat first (until almost done) crumble, and then add to the ingredients before baking.

Garlic Shrimp

Preheat oven to 350 degrees, 176.6C

Ingredients:

4 or more garlic cloves (I prefer to add more), thinly sliced
Red pepper to your liking for a little spice
1 dozen or more shrimp, depending on servings
½ cup or more olive oil to marinate the shrimp. This depends on how many servings you are making. Just make sure the shrimp is saturated.

Directions:

Place the shrimp in a bowl and add olive oil, the sliced garlic, red pepper and marinate for at least ½ hour or longer up to two hours. Spread the shrimp on a lined baking sheet along with the olive oil from the marinade (including the sliced garlic and red pepper flakes) poured over the shrimp. Bake at 350 degrees F for about 7 to 10 minutes or until done.

Coconut Rice

Bits of cauliflower enveloped in a toasted coconut milk and cardamom sauce. Coconut "rice" without the grains or starch.

Ingredients:

- 1 medium cauliflower or a bag or already riced cauliflower from Trader Joe's
- ⅓ cup finely diced white onion
- 3 tbsp. coconut oil
- ½ tsp. ground cardamom
- ¾ cup of full fat coconut milk in a can most markets carry this
- ¼ cup chopped cilantro
- A generous amount of salt and pepper

Directions:

Break the cauliflower into florets and either grate the florets with a cheese grater or buy it already riced from

Trader Joe's as mentioned above. You may also rice the cauliflower slowly in a blender pulsing it to get it into the rice form. Heat a large nonstick skillet over medium high heat for 1 to 2 minutes, add the coconut oil. Add the onion sauté until tender about five minutes. Then add the cardamom and stir with a wooden spoon until fragrant about 30 seconds. Add the rice and coconut milk stirring to combine for about 10 to 12 minutes until the coconut milk is absorbed. The consistency will be a little off for a while but it will come together as the cauliflower dries out a bit and brown specs begin to appear. Season with a generous amount of salt and pepper and add the ¼ cup chopped cilantro.

Note: I like to add the drippings from baking the shrimp into the rice.

Mango salsa (optional) but it truly does add to the taste

Ingredients:

> 2 semi ripe mangoes pitted, peeled and cut into small cubes
> 1 cup fresh cilantro chopped
> ½ medium red onion peeled or approximately ¾ of a cup chopped
> 1 jalapeño seeded
> 1 tbsp. lime juice or lemon juice
> ½ cucumber peeled cut into small cubes

Directions:

> Place all ingredients into a bowl mix and serve.

"Mock" Garlic Mashed Potatoes

Ingredients:

    1 medium head cauliflower
    ¼ cup (approx.) coconut milk
    ½ tsp. minced garlic or none
    ⅛ tsp. straight chicken base or bullion (may substitute
       ½ teaspoon salt)
    ½ tsp. freshly ground black pepper
    ½ tsp. chopped fresh or dry chives, for garnish
    3 to 4 tbsp. unsalted butter

Directions:

Set a stockpot of water to boil over high heat. Clean and cut cauliflower into small pieces. Cook in boiling water for about 6 minutes, or until well done. Drain well; do not let it cool, pat cooked cauliflower very dry between several layers of paper towels. In a bowl with an immersion blender, or in a regular blender or in a food processor, Puree the hot cauliflower with the garlic, chicken base, coconut milk and pepper until almost smooth. Garnish with chives, and serve hot with pats of butter.

REFERENCES

PART 3

The Obesity Epidemic and How We Got Wrong

1. Chowdhury R, Warnakula S, Kunutsor S, et al. Association of dietary, circulating, and supplement fatty acids with coronary risk; A systemic review. Ann Int Med. 2014;160(6):398-406.
2. Siri-Tarino PW, Sun Q, Hu FB, et al. Meta-analysis of prospective cohort studies evaluating the association of saturated fat with cardiovascular disease. Am J Clin Nutr. 2010;91(3):535-546.
3. Perlmutter D. Grain Brain. New York: Little, Brown and Co. 2013.
4. Davis W. Wheat Belly. New York: Rodale. 2011.
5. Jenkins, DJH, Wolever TM, Taylor RH, et al. Glycemic index of foods: a physiological basis for carbohydrate exchange. Am J Clin Nutr. 1981;34(3):362-366.
6. Juntunen KS, Niskanen LK, Liukkonen KH, et al. Postprandial glucose, insulin and incretin responses to grain products in healthy subjects. Am J Clin Nutr. 2002;75(2):254-262.
7. Jakobsen MU, Dethlefsen C, Joensen AM, at al. Intake of carbohydrates compared with intake of saturated fatty acids and the risk of myocardial infarction: Importance of the glycemic index. Am J Clin Nutr. 2010;91:1764-1768.

Does Gluten Cause Health Problems in Patients Without Celiac Disease?

1. Davis W. Wheat Belly. New York: Rodale, 2011.
2. Isasi C, Colmenero I, Casco F, et al. Fibromyalgia and non-celiac gluten sensitivity: a description with remission of fibromyalgia. Rheumatol Int. 2014;April 12 (Epub ahead of print).
3. Carroccio A, Volta U, Petrolini N, et al. Autoimmune enteropathy and colitis in an adult patient. Dig Dis Sci. 2003;48:1600-1606.
4. Volta U, De Giorgio. New understanding of gluten sensitivity. Nat Rev Gastroenterol Hepatol 2012;9:295-299.
5. Anonymous patient, Rostami K, Hogg-Kollars S, Non-coeliac gluten sensitivity. BMJ 2012;345:e7982.
6. Sapone A, Bai JC, Ciacci C, et al. Spectrum of gluten-related disorders: consensus on new nomenclature and classification. BMC Medicine 2012;10:13.
7. Isasi C, Fernandez-Puga N, Serrano-Vela JI. Fibromyalgia and chronic fatigue syndrome caused by non-celiac gluten sensitivity. Rheumatol Clin. 2014; July 18 (Epub ahead of print).
8. Hadjivassiliou M, Sanders DS, Grunewald RA, et al. Gluten sensitivity; from gut to brain. Lancet. 2010;9:318-330.
9. Perlmutter D, Grain Brain. New York; Little Brown, 2013.
10. Campbell TC, Jacobson H. Whole: Rethinking the Science of Nutrition. Dallas: BenBella, 2013.

Wheat Causes Intestinal Immune Activation in Some People Without Celiac Disease

1. Glenn JD, Mowry EM. Emerging Concepts on the Gut Microbiome and Multiple Sclerosis. Journal of Interferon & Cytokine Research. 2016;36(6):1-11.
2. Volta U, Bardella MT, Calabro A, Troncone R, Corazza GR, et al. An Italian prospective multicenter survey on patients suspected of having non-celiac gluten sensitivity. BMC Med. 2014;12:85.
3. Volta U, De Giorgio. New understanding of gluten sensitivity. Nat Rev Gastroenterol Hepatol 2012;9:295-299.
4. Perlmutter D, Loberg K. Grain Brain. New York: Little, Brown and Co. 2013.
5. Mullen G. The Gut Balance Revolution. New York: Rodale. 2015.
6. Wahls T. The Wahls Protocol. New York: Avery (Penguin Group), 2014.
7. http://www.brainyquote.com/quotes/quotes/m/m aimonides326756.html

PART 4

Profile in Courage – Robert Atkins

1. Quoted in Stevenson AE. Call to Greatness. Harper, 1954.
2. Bazzano LA, Hu T, Reynolds K, et al. Effects of Low-Carbohydrate and Low-Fat Diets: A

Randomized Trial. Ann Intern Med. 2014;161:309-318.

3. Chowdhury R, Warnakula S, Kunutsor S, et al. Association of dietary, circulating, and supplement fatty acids with coronary risk; A systemic review. Ann Int Med. 2014;160(6):398-406.

4. Siri-Tarino PW, Sun Q, Hu FB, et al. Meta-analysis of prospective cohort studies evaluating the association of saturated fat with cardiovascular disease. Am J Clin Nutr. 2010;91(3):535-546.

5. Volek JS, Phinney SD. The Art and Science of Low Carbohydrate Living. Beyond Obesity, LLC. 2011.

6. Jakobsen MU, Dethlefsen C, Joensen AM, at al. Intake of carbohydrates compared with intake of saturated fatty acids and the risk of myocardial infarction: Importance of the glycemic index. Am J Clin Nutr. 2010;91:1764-1768.

7. Davis W. Wheat Belly. Rodale. 2011.

8. Wikipedia, Robert Atkins. Accessed September 30, 2014.

9. Gordon ES, Goldberg M, Chosy GJ. A New Concept in the Treatment of Obesity. JAMA. 1963;186(1):156-166.

10. Atkins RC. Dr. Atkins' Diet Revolution. Bantam Books. 1972.

11. American Medical Association Council on Foods and Nutrition. A Critique of Low-Carbohydrate Ketogenic Weight Reduction Regimens: A Review of Dr. Atkins' Diet Revolution. JAMA. 1973;224:1415-1419.

12. Kuhn TS. The Structure of Scientific Revolutions. University of Chicago Press. 1962.

13. Volek JS, Phinney SD. The Art and Science of Low Carbohydrate Performance. Beyond Obesity, LLC. 2012.
14. Atkins RC. Dr. Atkins' New Diet Revolution. Harper. 1992, 1999, 2002.
15. Jenkins, DJH, Wolever TM, Taylor RH, et al. Glycemic index of foods: a physiological basis for carbohydrate exchange. Am J Clin Nutr. 1981;34(3):362-366.
16. Agatson A. The South Beach Diet. St. Martin's Press. 2003.
17. Voegtlin WL. The Stone Age Diet. Vantage Press, 1975.
18. Cordain L. The Paleo Diet. John Wiley & Sons, 2002, 2011.
19. Westman EC, Phinney SD, Volek JS. The New Atkins for a New You. Touchstone. 2010.
20. Willett WC. Eat, Drink, and Be Healthy: The Harvard Medical School Guide to Healthy Eating. Free Press. Simon & Schuster, 2005.
21. O'Connor A. A Call for a Low-Carb Diet That Embraces Fat. New York Times. September 1, 2014.
22. Perlmutter D. Grain Brain. Little, Brown and Co. 2013.
23. Warren R, Amen D, Hyman M. The Daniel Plan: 40 Days to a Healthier Life. Zondervan, 2013.
24. Townsend A. Cleveland Clinic to open Center for Functional Medicine; Dr. Mark Hyman to be director. Cleveland Plain Dealer. www.cleveland.com/healthfit/index.ssf/2014/09/cl eveland_clinic_to_open/cente.html.
25. Campbell TC, Jacobson H. Whole: Rethinking the Science of Nutrition. BenBella Books, 2013.

26. Forks Over Knives. Virgil Films Entertainment, 2011. www.youtube.com/user/ForksOverKnives

Overweight and Obesity – It's the Carbohydrates

1. Gayelord Hauser. Widipedia.org. Accessed February 5, 2015.
2. Gordon ES, Goldberg M, Chosy GJ. A New Concept in the Treatment of Obesity. JAMA. 1963;186(1):156-166.
3. Wikipedia, Robert Atkins. Accessed February 5, 2015.
4. Atkins RC. Dr. Atkins' Diet Revolution. Bantam Books. 1972.
5. Agatson A. The South Beach Diet. St. Martin's Press. 2003.
6. Bazzano LA, Hu T, Reynolds K, et al. Effects of Low-Carbohydrate and Low-Fat Diets: A Randomized Trial. Ann Intern Med. 2014;161:309-318.
7. Chowdhury R, Warnakula S, Kunutsor S, et al. Association of dietary, circulating, and supplement fatty acids with coronary risk; A systemic review. Ann Int Med. 2014;160(6):398-406.
8. Siri-Tarino PW, Sun Q, Hu FB, et al. Meta-analysis of prospective cohort studies evaluating the association of saturated fat with cardiovascular disease. Am J Clin Nutr. 2010;91(3):535-546.
9. Volek JS, Phinney SD. The Art and Science of Low Carbohydrate Living. Beyond Obesity, LLC. 2011.
10. Jakobsen MU, Dethlefsen C, Joensen AM, at al. Intake of carbohydrates compared with intake of saturated fatty acids and the risk of myocardial

infarction: Importance of the glycemic index. Am J Clin Nutr. 2010;91:1764-1768.

11. Volek JS, Phinney SD. The Art and Science of Low Carbohydrate Performance. Beyond Obesity, LLC. 2012.

12. Davis W. Wheat Belly. Rodale. 2011.

13. Campbell TC, Jacobson H. Whole: Rethinking the Science of Nutrition. BenBella Books, 2013.

14. Minger D. Death By Food Pyramid. Primal Blueprint Publishing, 2013.

15. Voegtlin WL. The Stone Age Diet. Vantage Press, 1975.

16. Cordain L. The Paleo Diet. John Wiley & Sons, 2002, 2011.

17. Dukan Diet. Wikipedia.org, Accessed February 18, 2015.

18. Davis W. Wheat Belly Total Health, Rodale, 2014.

19. Perlmutter D. Grain Brain. Little, Brown and Co. 2013.

20. Townsend A. Cleveland Clinic to open Center for Functional Medicine; Dr. Mark Hyman to be director. Cleveland Plain Dealer. www.cleveland.com/healthfit/index.ssf/2014/09/cl eveland_clinic_to_open/cente.html

21. Kuhn TS. The Structure of Scientific Revolutions. University of Chicago Press. 1962.

PART 5

Wheat Belly Total Health

1. Davis W. *Wheat Belly*. New York:Rodale, 2011.

2. Institute for Functional Medicine.
    www.functionalmedicine.org
3. Bazzano LA, Hu T, Reynolds K, et al. Effects of Low-Carbohydrate and Low-Fat Diets: A Randomized Trial. Ann Intern Med. 2014;161:309-318.
4. Hadjivassiliou M, Sanders DS, Grunewald RA, et al. Gluten sensitivity; from gut to brain. Lancet. 2010;9:318-330.
5. Volta U, Bardella MT, Calabro A, Troncone R, Corazza GR, et al. An Italian prospective multicenter survey on patients suspected of having non-celiac gluten sensitivity. BMC Med. 2014;12:85.
6. Perlmutter D. Grain Brain. New York: Little, Brown & Co., 2013.
7. Perlmutter D, Loberg K. Brain Maker. New York: Little, Brown & Co. 2015.
8. Hyman M. The Blood Sugar Solution 10 Day Detox Diet. New York: Little, Brown & Co. 2014.

Brain Maker

1. NIH Human Microbiome Project.
    http://hmpdacc.org/
2. Smith PA. Can the Bacteria in Your Gut Explain Your Mood? New York Times, June 23, 2015.

You Are What You Feed Your Gut Microbiome

1. Galland L. The gut microbiome and the brain. J Med Food. 2014;17:1261-1272.

2. O'Mahony SM, Clarke G, Borre YE, Dinan TG, Cryan JF. Serotonin, tryptophan metabolism and the brain-gut-microbiome axis. Behavioural Brain Research. 2015;277:32-48.

3. Perlmutter D. Brain Maker. New York: Little, Brown and Co. 2015.

4. Mayer EA, Tillisch K, Gupta A. Gut/brain axis and the microbiota. J. Clin Invest. 2015;125:926-938.

5. NIH Human Microbiome Project. http://hmpdacc.org/

The Wahls Protocol

1. http://terrywahls.com

Does Dysbiosis Cause Multiple Sclerosis?

1. Neu J, Rushing J. Cesarean versus vaginal delivery: long-term infant outcomes and the hygiene hypothesis. Clin Perinatol. 2011;38:321-331.

2. Pisacane A, Impagliazzo N, Russo M, et al. Breastfeeding and multiple sclerosis. J Leukoc Biol. 1994;308:1411-1412.

3. Lepage P, Colombet J, Marteau P, et al. Dysbiosis in inflammatory bowel disease: a role for bacteriophages? Gut. 2008;57:424-425.

4. Cantarel BL, Waubant E, Chehoud C, et al. Gut microbiota in multiple sclerosis: possible influence of immunomodulators. J Investig Med. 2015;63:729-734.

5. Perlmutter D. Brain Maker. New York: Little, Brown and Co. 2015.

6. Chutkin R. The Microbiome Solution. New York: Avery (Penguin). 2015.

7. Sonnenburg J, Sonnenburg E. The Good Gut. New York: Penguin Press. 2015.

8. Mullen G. The Gut Balance Revolution. New York: Rodale. 2015.

9. Wahls T. The Wahls Protocol. New York: Avery (Penguin Group), 2014.

Eat Fat, Get Thin

1. Hyman M. The Blood Sugar Solution. New York: Little, Brown and Co. 2012.

2. Perlmutter D, Loberg K. Grain Brain. New York: Little, Brown and Co. 2013.

3. Mullen G. The Gut Balance Revolution. New York: Rodale. 2015.

4. Wahls T. The Wahls Protocol. New York: Avery (Penguin Group), 2014.

5. Hamdy O. Nutrition revolution – the end of the high carbohydrates era for diabetes prevention and management. US Endocrinol. 2014;10(2)103-104.

6. Ludwig D. Always Hungry? New York: Hachette Book Group, 2016.

Welcome Back, Saturated Fat

1. Executive Committee on Diet and Heart Disease. *National Diet-Heart Study Report.* American Heart Association, 1968.
2. Getz GS, Vesselinovitch D, Wissler RW. A dynamic pathology of arteriosclerosis. Am J Med. 1969;46:657-673.
3. Oh K, Hu FB, Manson JE, et al. Dietary fat intake and risk of coronary heart disease in women: 20 years of follow-up of the nurses' health study. Am J Epidemiol. 2005;161:672-679.
4. Ramsden CE, Zamora D, Leelarthaepin B, et al. Use of dietary linoleic acid for secondary prevention of coronary heart disease and death: evaluation of recovered data from the Sydney Diet Heart Study and updated meta-analysis. BMJ. 2013;346:e8707.
5. Hyman M. Eat Fat, Get Thin: Why the Fat We Eat is the Key to Sustained Weight Loss and Vibrant Health. New York: Little, Brown and Company, 2016.
6. Bazzano LA, Hu T, Reynolds K, et al. Effects of Low-Carbohydrate and Low-Fat Diets: A Randomized Trial. Ann Intern Med. 2014;161:309-318.

ABOUT THE AUTHOR

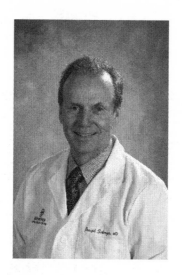

Joseph E. Scherger, M.D., M.P.H., is Vice President for Primary Care and Marie E. Pinizzotto, MD, Chair of Academic Affairs at Eisenhower Medical Center in Rancho Mirage, California. Dr. Scherger is President of the Riverside County Medical Association (RCMA) in 2017. He is also a Clinical Professor of Family Medicine at the Keck School of Medicine at the University of Southern California (USC). Dr. Scherger is a leader in transforming office practice and has special interests in nutrition and wellness. He has authored and self-published two previous books on Amazon, *40 Years in Family Medicine (2014),* and the first edition of *Lean and Fit* (2016).

Originally from Delphos, Ohio, Dr. Scherger graduated from the University of Dayton in 1971, summa cum laude. He graduated from the UCLA School of Medicine in 1975, and was elected to Alpha Omega Alpha. He completed a Family Medicine Residency and a Masters in Public Health at the University of Washington in 1978. From 1978-80, he served in the National Health Service Corps in Dixon, California, as a migrant health physician. From 1981-92, Dr. Scherger divided his time between private practice in Dixon and teaching medical students and residents at UC Davis. From 1988-91, he was a Fellow in the Kellogg National Fellowship Program, focusing on health care reform and quality of life. From 1992-1996, he was Vice President for Family Practice and Primary Care Education at Sharp HealthCare in San Diego. From 1996-2001, he was the Chair of the Department of Family Medicine and the Associate Dean for Primary Care at the University of California Irvine. From 2001-2003, Dr. Scherger served as founding dean of the Florida State University College of Medicine.

Dr. Scherger has received numerous awards, including being recognized as a "Top Doc" in San Diego for 6 consecutive years, 2004-2009. He was voted Outstanding Clinical Instructor at the University of California, Davis School of Medicine in 1984, 1989 and 1990. In 1989, he was Family Physician of the Year by the American Academy of Family Physicians and the California Academy of Family Physicians. In 1986, he was President of the Society of Teachers of Family Medicine. In 1992, Dr. Scherger was elected to the Institute of Medicine of the National Academy of Sciences. In 1994, he received the Thomas W. Johnson Award for Family Practice Education from the American Academy of Family Physicians. In 2000, he was selected by the UC Irvine medical students for the

AAMC Humanism in Medicine Award. He received the Lynn and Joan Carmichael Recognition Award from the Society of Teachers of Family Medicine in 2012. He served on the Institute of Medicine Committee on the Quality of Health Care in America from 1998-2001. Dr. Scherger served on the Board of Directors of the American Academy of Family Physicians and the American Board of Family Medicine. From 2005-2010 he served as Consulting Medical Director for Quality and Informatics at Lumetra Healthcare Solutions.

Dr. Scherger serves on the editorial board of *Medical Economics* and is an Assistant Editor of *Family Medicine*. He is a Senior Fellow with the Estes Park Institute. He was the Men's Health expert and a consultant for Revolution Health, 2006-09, and he has covered California for eDocAmerica since 2003. He was Editor-in-Chief of *Hippocrates*, published by the Massachusetts Medical Society, from 1999-2001. He was the first Medical Editor of *Family Practice Management.* He has authored more than 400 medical publications and has given over 1000 invited presentations.

Dr. Scherger enjoys an active family life with his wife, Carol, and two sons, Adrian and Gabriel. He has completed 37 marathons, ten 50K and five 50 mile ultramarathon trail runs.